BLOODLETTING
TO BINARY

A Physician
A Small Hospital in Rhode Island
An Extraordinary Era in American Medicine

E. B. McKee, M.D.

Publisher's Information

EBookBakery Books

Author contact: michael@ebookbakery.com

ISBN 978-1-938517-63-1

1. Medical. 2. Memoir. 3. History 4. South County Rhode Island.

© 2016 by E. B. McKee, M.D.

ACKNOWLEDGMENTS

Essential to the narrative were those who gave generously of their time and recollections. The list includes Doctors Joseph O'Neill, Tim Drury, Larry Bouchard, Bob Conrad (and wife Marty), Kenneth Hathaway, John O'Leary, James Murdocco, and Jack Cooke, physician's assistant. John Miller, a Narragansett native, provided valuable historical insight.

My wife Pat, as a major player in the memoir, offered her recollections (sometimes at variance with mine), while restraining my inclination to hyperbole.

Tracy Hart provided her usual impeccable editorial expertise; Michael Grossman shepherded the manuscript through the publishing process during which his infinite patience was regularly tested.

DEDICATION

*To the physicians, nurses and other medical providers
I have worked with through the years.*

BLOODLETTING
TO BINARY

TABLE OF CONTENTS

- PREFACE -

In 2013, I wrote a memoir (*DOC*), which traced the circuitous route I – a recent college graduate – followed in search of a medical school which would accept me. The quest stretched to Ireland, England, Scotland, and France. The conflict in the tale related to two factors: my complete disinterest in medicine, and the determination of a formidable aunt who insisted I become a physician. Mainly to placate her, while imagining a couple of months of travel as great fun, I set off. The memoir recounted the search, my acceptance at the Royal College of Surgeons in Dublin, the years in Ireland, my eventual graduation, and subsequent return to the United Sates to launch my career.

My aversion to the sciences (and medicine as a future occupation), persisted through my first two years of medical school. My motivation for exam success: it allowed me to stay in school so I could continue to enjoy life in Ireland. For the first time in memory I had no one to answer to; I embraced my liberation enthusiastically.

It was during the clinical years, when the connection between book and bedside was demonstrated on a daily basis that a semblance of interest took hold. The banter between an attending and his retinue, as they made their way through a thicket of competing pathologies to establish a diagnosis and treatment plan, stirred a curiosity. I was well removed from that ability, but deciding to acquire the necessary tools was a notable step forward. The good times continued, but a dash of purpose had been added to the mix. By the time of my graduation I couldn't imagine being involved in any other profession.

The recollections in (*Bloodletting to Binary*) pick up where *DOC* left off, with the exception of a gap between 1961 and 1963: my internship and residency years at Memorial Hospital in Pawtucket R.I. The mishaps, humbling experiences, successes, and short-lived romances remain an amorphous blur. My most persistent memory: being chronically tired and feeling poorly the last six months of the training. So rather than subject the reader to my laments, I felt it best to set those days aside.

Divided into two parts, I first write about the period prior to my return to Rhode Island (including three years of active duty with the Air Force, and post-discharge, my employment with United Airlines). The second section begins with my private practice getting underway in South County and finishes with my retirement. My focus is on the early years, particularly the 1960's and 1970's, when the face of medicine – how it was practiced and paid for – dramatically changed. South County Hospital was a microcosm of this transition.

Physicians, hospital activities, and personnel from that period receive the most attention. The staff (physicians and nurses), was small enough to allow an easy familiarity which I have tried to illustrate in my narrative. The decades that followed were marked by an explosion in medical staff membership and hospital services. Rather than attempt what certainly would be an inadequate portrayal of those days, I have limited the scope to the people and times I knew best.

Nurses are not mentioned by name. This in no way reflects a lack of regard. No physician has appreciated their talents more than I. They have saved my tail and had my back on occasions too numerous to remember. So frequent, in fact, that rather than chance an embarrassing exclusion, they remain anonymous. But they know who they are.

Incidents and stories related in this book are as recalled by me. Others may have a different version, but to the extent possible, I have verified (either by interview or research), the correctness of my account. The dialogue in many instances does not contain the precise verbiage used at the time, but the tone and intent of the conversations are depicted accurately. In many instances, names and details have been altered to discourage identification. One of the benefits of doing a memoir at this stage of life: many of whom you write are no longer around to defend themselves.

This memoir is an abridged rendering, more sunshine than shadow. The unabridged narrative will have to wait until some kindly physician tells me I have six months remaining on the planet; if that dour diagnosis is confirmed with a second opinion – I will set about penning a more purple prose. Until then I hope you will enjoy the sepia-tinged recollections of this physician's journey, meeting some of his companions along the way, gaining a sense of an extraordinary time.

Gene McKee
November, 2016

INTRODUCTION

We were making good time. The 1964 Nash Rambler, unused to lengthy excursions, was performing admirably. Clear of New Haven's clutter, a sign indicated Old Saybrook, Connecticut, thirty miles away. I mentioned our respectable progress to my wife, Pat, who nodded in agreement.

"At this rate," she said, "we should be there by early afternoon."

"There" was Wakefield, Rhode Island and on this May morning in 1970, the destination of the McKee family.

The trip had begun the previous day in Massapequa, New York, a small community on Long Island's south coast. After a stop at Kennedy Airport, where I had been employed by United Airlines (UAL), we joined the stream of cars crossing the Throgs Neck Bridge into Connecticut. The weather, inclement to start, rapidly worsened as afternoon darkened into evening. Thunder, lightning, and a slashing rain overwhelmed the car's windshield wipers, forcing refuge in a West Haven motel. Safe from the storm raging outside, we had a pleasant supper and except for a daughter who used the crib as a trampoline for what seemed half the night, enjoyed a refreshing sleep.

As is often the case after a night of violent weather, the morning was spectacular: vivid blue sky, an occasional blemish of cloud, air fresh and clean, a warming sun. After breakfast and some luggage adjustments, we were back on the freeway, the traffic meager that early Saturday morning. The roads were drying out. Water skimmed along the gutters, puddles collected at the runoffs; grass borders were matted flat from car spray, and glistening tree branches bent with moisture.

On this optimistic spring morning, I was in my thirty-sixth year. My premature acquisition of gray hair led many who met me to inflate that number. Pat, although within shouting distance of my age, looked years younger – a "delicate beauty," as she was once described. This fortunate attribute caused many to think her my daughter, to my chagrin.

In the back seat, squeezed between clothes, boxes, and an awkwardly placed plant, were three children: Matthew, a fair-haired boy of four, presently following our progress on his map; and his sisters, one-year-old Ellen, quietly coloring; and five-month-old Katy, sleeping.

Since time was not a constraint, we decided to follow Route 1 between New Haven and New London. Although less direct than the freeway, on previous trips we had found it a particularly picturesque stretch. Following the coastline, we looped around small villages tucked into the shore, marinas crowded with power boats, sailboats in secluded coves, the first blooms of rhododendrons, and on occasion, a glittering Long Island Sound.

Remarking on the benevolent weather, Pat wondered if I was aware of the superstition which claims a stormy day to be an omen that bodes well for whatever project is begun on such a dismal day.

"For sure," I replied. "Anything begun in the rain is a shoo-in to succeed, sort of like a baptism. Especially marriages. A little soaking on that day just about guarantees a long run."

"Too bad today is such a nice day, with our big move and everything," Pat said.

"It rained through the early morning. The ground is still wet. I think we're covered."

"I hope so."

"Me too."

The decision to uproot the family and head north had achieved consensus after much thought and discussion of the options. Three hours a day on the Long Island Expressway provided a daily dose of tedium, but the commute itself was not a game changer. My job at the airport paid an adequate wage with excellent benefits, but offered little challenge. Hence, my primary concerns were: forsaking the security of a stable company, entering the ranks of the self-employed, and making enough money to support the family. Our savings, I estimated, would cover us for approximately three months.

There are moments, however, in everyone's life when deep down you know it's time to move on: an itch that needs to be scratched, a decision made, a chance taken. And this was one of them. Although my situation was not as dire as Farragut's "Damn the torpedoes, full speed ahead" experience, it expressed my sentiment at the time. Also, as a Rhode Island kid, my family spent summers in Narragansett, a town adjacent to Wakefield, and I always had a hankering to return.

Meanwhile, Pat's concerns were more domestic: settling into a partially furnished home, school for Matthew, available playmates, church affiliations, fitting into the community.

A rest area after New London gave everyone a chance to move about (especially the kids, immobilized for two hours), enjoy a snack, and relieve bladder concerns.

Thirty minutes later, our surprisingly durable Rambler chugged into Rhode Island. In something of a victory lap, we confidently followed a winding country road past two golf courses, a train station, and the entrance to the University of Rhode Island. We arrived in Wakefield, a comfortable stretch of commercial activity divided into two parts by a single road, presently under repair.

The look of the town had changed little since I was a kid. The red brick mill complex, sprawled by the weir on the Pettaquamscutt River, remained but appeared unoccupied. Along Main Street, the car dealership, grocery store, Sheldon's Home Furnishings, Kenyon's department store, and DiFanti's Pharmacy stood as before. A turn by the Episcopal Church brought us along tree-lined Kenyon Avenue and its parade of fine, older residences. Finally, we turned onto Hillcrest Road and pointed out our new home to a couple of excited kids. (Katy didn't seem impressed.)

The moving van carrying our furniture was scheduled to arrive by midafternoon. In fact, it arrived about 5:30. From the outset, the tone of voice and body language of the two moving men screamed belligerence. Their journey had been slowed, they said, by inaccurate directions that took over an hour to correct. The prospect of returning to New York later than planned was probably the reason for their irritability. Pat later told me she could smell alcohol.

"Before we can unload your stuff," said the driver, who was the older of the two, "we need a check for five hundred dollars." I dug my checkbook from the glove compartment, filled in the amount, and handed it to the driver.

"No, Mister," he said, "this won't do. Gotta be a bank check or cash."

"Look," I said, "I don't have that kind of cash with me, and all the banks are closed."

"Then we don't move you. Simple as that."

They gave the impression that they would like to turn their rig around and head back to New York, postponing the two or so hours of unloading until another day.

Pat was beyond angry. Her eyes glinted of violence.

I asked the driver to call his boss so I could speak with him.

"Nope, can't do that," he said. "Warehouse's closed."

Pat began arguing with both men. The younger of the two climbed into the cab and lit a cigarette. Not a good moment. The kids were getting antsy. The excitement of running through the new house had worn off. The baby was due a feeding. Everyone was hungry and tired.

A thought occurred: *Maybe a local pharmacy will cash a check.*

"OK," I said to the driver, "let's see what I can do."

"You've got a half hour, Mister. Not back by then, we're taking off."

The small lady behind the counter at the South County Pharmacy had a pleasant voice, neatly coiffed hair, and kind eyes behind dark-rimmed glasses. She came from behind the tall counter at the rear of the store to the checkout counter where I was standing. There was no one else in the place.

"Hello," she said. "What can I do for you?"

I explained the situation and added, "I'm a new physician coming into town. I'd really appreciate it if you would cash a check for me."

She looked at me closely, scanning my jeans, T-shirt, sneakers. I sensed her hesitation.

"Have your license?" she asked.

"Yes, but not with me. I didn't think I'd be needing it."

She gave me a puzzled look, then smiled. "No, not your medical one. Your driver's license." She looked at it briefly and handed it back. "Where's your office going to be?"

"Medical building by the Narragansett rotary."

She paused for a moment, tidying the counter as she considered my request.

"Okay," she finally said, "make out the check to South County Pharmacy." She walked behind the tall counter and exited through a back door.

A few minutes later, she returned with a paper bag, the contents of which she dumped on the counter. A mound of cash. Most of the bills were in packets bound by elastic, the others loose and wrinkled. She separated them by denomination and added them up. When she reached $500, she stopped and handed the bills to me.

"I can't tell you how appreciative I am –"

She waved me off. "Welcome to town, Dr. McKee."

So on May 26, 1970, I gratefully accepted the welcome and extraordinary kindness of Mary Tafuri, pharmacist and owner of the South County Pharmacy.

It was after midnight when we called it a day, the first floor still strewn with boxes, furniture, clothes, utensils. Pat (organized and uncomfortable with disarray), agreed with reluctance. The kids were asleep, their bellies full, the house cozy on a chilly night, every utility that should work did. A long day ending well.

"The rest can wait," I told her. "Won't look so bad in the morning."

Pat plopped into a lounge chair. Clearing some space, I stretched out on a couch, whose legs had yet to be found. We split – unequally – a bottle of beer found in an otherwise empty refrigerator. We toasted to the first night in our new home.

"Never again," Pat announced.

"Never again what?" I asked.

"This is our last move."

"Agreed," I answered, "this time we settle and stay."

"I've heard that line before. But this time I mean it." Her voice was raspy, eyes heavy, face full of tired. "We've been on the road three years, three states, three kids." Quiet for a moment, she sipped her beer. "But it was probably good to get it out of our system." Then she added, "Make it easier to settle down."

"It's been a long haul. But like you said, I think we're ready. A new chapter about to begin. Sort of curious how it's all going to turn out."

"Okay, Captain," she said, yawning, "while you're being curious I'm going to bed."

Halfway up the stairs, she stopped and turned. "I also wonder how the story will end."

I didn't respond as I didn't know the answer. But I certainly remembered how it began.

I finished her beer, turned off the lights, and followed her up the stairs.

- PART ONE -

AIR FORCE DAYS

In 1963, after completing my internship and residency in family medicine at Memorial Hospital in Pawtucket, Rhode Island, I entered the Air Force. It was payback time for an ROTC commitment from college days.

My three years in the hospital had taken their toll. The thirty-hours-on and twelve-hours-off schedule had whittled my weight down from 165 to 140 pounds. Nausea and appetite loss were persistent concerns. The occasional beer or two I hoisted on an evening off triggered vomiting, a situation which persisted for months. The checks I received every two weeks from the hospital were stashed in a drawer, no time to spend them. In some ways, my entrance into the military was a lifesaver.

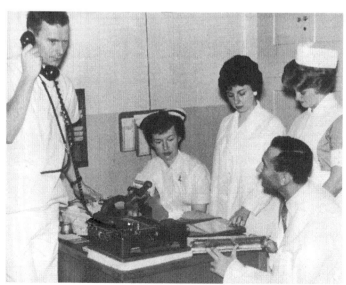

Dr. McKee with fellow physician and Memorial Hospital personnel, 1962

Conversations with Air Force personnel prior to my entrance into active duty assured me that every effort would be made to honor my requests for duty assignments. With that in mind, bases in Hawaii, the Far East, and various European locations were chosen. Finally, I thought, a chance to break away, discard the familiar and experience those "faraway places with strange-sounding names." With great anticipation I tore open the official letter that would inform me of the base I would call home for the next three years.

"Congratulations," it began. "You have been assigned to 551st USAF Wing, Otis Air Force Base, Cape Cod, Massachusetts." The base was approximately one hour from the spot where I was standing at that moment.

I arrived at Otis on the appointed day and designated time. To my surprise, I had been assigned to the Base Supply Squadron. This caused some merriment among the members of that unit; there was general agreement that the outfit needed medical help, the pity being I wasn't a psychiatrist. The paperwork was quickly amended, transferring me to the hospital roster.

General medical officer became my title; I was assigned to the pediatric service. Uniforms were purchased at base clothing, and a sergeant working in administration took me aside and demonstrated a crisp salute and the proper placement of insignias on my uniform.

Twelve other physicians completed the medical staff. Most had finished their residencies and were fulfilling ROTC or other government obligations, as I was. Two were military career doctors: Dr. Paul Stavig, Hospital Commander, and Dr. Len Cobb, an obstetrician.

The chief of pediatrics, whom I'd be working with, was Dr. Ed Jablonski, board-certified two months earlier. He'd received his training at Boston Children's Hospital. From the outset we got along well, although I thought his insistence that morning rounds be conducted at 6:30 a.m. was particularly uncivilized. His reason: he wanted the night nurse's report directly, concerned that the day nurse might omit some of the details. Besides being very knowledgeable, Dr. Jablonski was meticulous and compulsive, traits any mother would be pleased to discover in her baby's physician.

Over the course of the next few weeks, between staff meetings, cafeteria interactions, and chats over coffee, the heretofore homogenous staff began to separate out. Individuals emerged, distinguished by personality, temperament, and idiosyncrasy. With this particular group, I was struck by how closely some of its members conformed to the persona associated with their specialties:

The Caring Pediatrician

At ease with both children and mothers, Dr. Jablonski addressed their concerns with understanding and skill. After observing his infinite patience with mothers and his ability to establish rapport with youngsters – two traits clearly necessary in that specialty – the inclination I had to pursue a pediatric residency was set aside.

The Cocky, Aggressive Surgeon

Two years removed from his residency at a prestigious New York hospital, one of our two surgeons was the poster boy for the cocky, instrument-flinging, tantrum-prone Grand Pooh-Bah of the operating room. Questions by patients relative to a proposed surgery were batted away with "the nurse will explain all that to you." To his credit, he was an excellent surgeon with consistently good results.

Some months later, though, his hubris became his undoing. He undertook a thoracic surgery beyond his capability and which exceeded the resources of our facility, in terms of both personnel and equipment. The patient, a pilot in his mid-forties, died on the operating table. The doctor's surgical privileges were curtailed, and a peer review followed. A short time later he was separated from the military.

The Kindly Obstetrician

Relaxing in the nurses' station after a delivery, chair tilted back, feet up, gray hair tousled, face friendly and florid, surgical mask dangling from one ear, pipe lit – an image crying out for Norman Rockwell – was Dr. Cobb.

The Studious Internist

Two were assigned to the hospital. Similar in appearance – medium height, lean stature, pale complexion, and each with horn-rimmed glasses – they shared an intellectual approach to patient care. The tactile portion of their care they tended to avoid. For them, the abdomen ended at the umbilicus, the expanse of flesh below seldom explored; surgical consults were requested for rectal exams. They seemed most at ease hunched behind a stack of cardiograms – they did all the EKG readings – reviewing X-rays or combing through medical journals.

To be fair, both were getting ready for the internal medicine boards, which required significant preparation. Their consults were impressive: thorough, well written, and replete with references supporting their recommendations. Though they were friendly and always available for questions relating to medications, diagnosis, and treatment, one sensed that they felt their time and talents were being wasted in the military milieu.

The Eccentric Psychiatrist

Dr. Tom worked out of a small office at the rear of the facility. His waiting room contained three chairs and a small table. There were no windows in either room. Patients entered through an unmarked back door. Dr. Tom lived off base, and with the exception of the occasional staff meeting, was seldom seen in the hospital proper. That probably suited the hospital commander just fine. Tom's long hair and beard, unkempt by military standards, and a uniform with that slept-in look, didn't reflect the image Dr. Stavig wished for his physicians.

When Tom did make an appearance, he was a lively presence. His endless supply of raunchy jokes and spot-on ethnic accents even had Dr. Stavig laughing out loud. Otherwise, Tom was a remote figure in the facility, a shadow that flitted in and out, barely glimpsed for weeks at a time.

My bias, admittedly unfair, was that many who entered the mental health profession – particularly in the psychology and counseling areas – did so to address and correct their own issues. The basis for this belief was totally anecdotal, solely a result of observation over a limited period of time.

A few years later, I discussed my perception with a psychiatrist in Denver. He agreed. "And they're successful," he added. "After an emotional connection has been established with the client, they transfer – often unconsciously – their own needs, their own problems to the patient. Counter-transference, it's called. The kicker is, as their client starts to improve, they begin to feel better themselves."

An interesting anecdote regarding Tom in his role as base psychiatrist: A young airman whose aggressive behavior on multiple occasions had resulted in significant injury to others in his unit, was referred to mental health for evaluation and fitness for duty. The airman was accompanied to the appointment by a military policeman (MP). While the patient was filling out the slew of forms prior to his interview, Tom chatted with the MP for perhaps fifteen minutes. After evaluation of the airman, he was returned to his holding cell.

Three days later, Tom's evaluation was received by the base commander. The conclusions: the airman involved in the altercations was mentally sound. His actions, the report said, were an acting-out mechanism, an adolescent response to authority. A series of follow-up visits was suggested and an eventual return to regular duties predicted.

There was an addendum. The MP who accompanied the airman, it stated, exhibited signs of deep-seated hostility which, if not checked, could manifest as violent behavior. It was further suggested that the MP not be allowed to carry firearms, with consideration given to removing him from his present assignment.

The MP, it was reported, was stunned. He had been five years in the security field with an unblemished record. What his eventual disposition was I never learned.

A small number of our hospital physicians had simmering attitude problems. They didn't want to be in the military, and although their opinions were not expressed publicly, their hostility was apparent. They came across as arrogant, condescending, and dismissive of the care offered in the facility, and looked ahead to the day when they could remove their uniforms, scrap the structure and regulations of the military, and return to civilian facilities, resources, and remuneration.

Patient care, it should be noted, was not adversely affected by their unfortunate sentiments. Unfortunate because, as I came to learn, the quality of care throughout the hospital was excellent. The surroundings may have left something to be desired, but patient satisfaction and outcomes were consistent with those of civilian facilities. Visitors from the Joint Commission on Accreditation of Healthcare Organizations (JCAHO) found little to fault during their inspections.

Roommates to Remember

Located within walking distance of the officers' club was the BOQ (Bachelor Officer Quarters), a square brick structure with accommodations for twenty-five single officers. Each suite included bathroom, two bedrooms, kitchenette, and living/dining room. During my first year there, I had two roommates.

The first, Vinny Castle (name altered), was a twenty-one-year-old pilot who had just returned from a Vietnam tour and had already signed up for a second. Short – about five feet six inches – and stocky with a buzz cut, Vinny embodied the gung-ho attitude, totally accepting and enthusiastically supporting the military mission in Southeast Asia, as I did. This was in 1963, years before the body bags, the Tet offensive, and the anti-war demonstrations, a time when American troops were designated "military advisors."

In Vietnam, Vinny was a FAC (forward air controller). Flying a light airplane over enemy territory at slow speed and low altitude (an extremely dangerous occupation), he sought out and tracked enemy troop movements and identified villages suspected of harboring Viet Cong. Having marked the areas with smoke grenades, he called in South Vietnamese aircraft for napalm strikes. Many villages, it turned out, housed only peasants. The "collateral" deaths of innocent people and the decimation of their villages was of little concern to Vinny.

"If they're yellow, I kill 'em," was his mantra. "They're all the same to me."

"No regrets?" I said. "You know, women and kids."

"Hell, no. That's what I do for a living. And," he added, "know what really makes my day?" He grinned. "A whole bunch of 'em running through the village, lit up like firecrackers. I waggle my wings and give them a wave."

Pretty callous stuff. But it was the way he was trained to think. No emotion. Mistakes are made. Innocent people get killed. That's war. And its guys like Vinny who win them for you.

He hung out socially with other pilots in his squadron. Occasionally, when he returned to the room after a night out with his buddies, he would load up his service revolver, turn up the volume on the TV, and fire at a tree stump he had set up at the end of the corridor in our quarters. Not wishing to be the recipient of a stray bullet, we had a conversation. A compromise was reached. No gun play while I was in-house. What he did in my absence was up to him.

Over the months I learned something of his background. He was the youngest of three, with two older sisters. To his frustration and the chagrin of his ex-athlete father, he never made it in sports – too light for football, too small for basketball, too slow for track. Nor did he make much of an impression on the girls; he took a cousin to his junior prom.

Then Vinny discovered the USAF. Blessed with intelligence and good eyesight, he qualified for flight school, earned his wings, and became a pilot – "the greatest accomplishment of my life." With it came confidence and self-esteem. No longer sitting on the sidelines, Vinny was playing with the big boys now. He couldn't wait to return to Vietnam and get back to work, calling in the jets, the power of life and death in his hands. "If my old man could see me now," he often said. Thrust into a position of authority for the first time in his life – a little man with a big gun – Vinny had found his niche, a dynamic often seen in law enforcement.

After about six months at Otis, Vinny was transferred to a base on the West Coast for refresher training prior to his return to Southeast Asia.

My next roommate, Aaron, was a dentist with a personality the polar opposite of Vinny. A smallish man with thinning black hair and a pale, timid face, he appeared to be in his early thirties. During our initial chat, he mentioned two things he felt I should be aware of "just to clear the air."

"I'm Jewish," he said. "And I'm gay. Will this be a problem?" He sounded apologetic.

"Can't imagine why it would," I answered, laughing. "I thought all dentists were Jewish. As for the other, if you're worried about privacy, we can work something out."

"That won't be a problem. My partner's in New York. We've been together for a few years, and that's not going to change."

Quiet, with a self-deprecating sense of humor and the ability to produce palatable meals from a stove which, to my knowledge, had never been used, Aaron became the ideal roomie. An extensive classical record collection replaced the saccharine sounds of Boone, Sinatra, and the Beach Boys. Magazines related to the theater, ballet, and the arts, neatly stacked on the coffee table, took precedence over the Playboy-type glossies formerly strewn about the place. Fastidious himself – the sign of a good dentist – the apartment took on a tidy and organized look. A plant now sat on the bullet-riddled tree stump in the hallway.

His undoing was perhaps inevitable considering his hormonal inclination and patient demographic. He was assigned to the F-101 fighter interceptor group, a macho bunch in their orange flight suits (more visible in case of ejection over water), caps at a jaunty angle, and a swagger in their step. They were generally fit and decent-looking – the '60s version of *The Right Stuff*. Apparently, while attending to their dental needs, Aaron found it difficult to keep his hands away from them, frequently having to recover instruments which had inadvertently fallen into their laps. Complaints were made; Aaron was referred to the base psychiatrist for evaluation.

Returning from a weekend away, I found the apartment empty of his things. "Enjoyed rooming with you," his note said. "Good luck with your career. Aaron."

The Camelot Connection

At regular intervals, Dr. Paul Stavig, the hospital commander, invited local specialists to speak at our staff meetings. One invitee was Janet Travell, MD, President Kennedy's personal physician since 1960. He frequently brought her along to Hyannisport, the summer White House. The president's back difficulties–sequelae of a failed discectomy and laminectomy –were well-documented, and Dr. Travell's treatments were successful in alleviating his discomfort. She championed the concept of "trigger points": small, tender areas in muscle which, when irritated, refer pain to surrounding areas. Once identified, they were injected with procaine, a local anesthetic, and the overlying skin sprayed with a coolant or xylocaine. Specific exercises were also prescribed and in the president's case, a rocking chair. Her talks and demonstrations of technique were informative, spiced with humor and the occasional Washington insider tale.

One of the benefits of her association with our hospital: invitations for single physicians to attend social functions, usually evening parties, at the compound in Hyannisport. Young women without partners were often in attendance; the physicians were brought in to chat, socialize, and otherwise relieve their solitary status.

One afternoon Dr. Stavig called to inform me that I was one of three physicians chosen to attend an event at the compound that evening – my first invite. Unfortunately, a cruel fate, in the guise of our oral surgeon, intervened; two of my wisdom teeth had been extracted that morning. My face was swollen, chipmunk fashion, my mind clouded with narcotic pain relief. With huge regret I declined. In the years since, flashes of fantasy have surfaced, visions of what might have been – perhaps an eager duchess endowed with a significant dowry, looking for her duke – if I hadn't missed my Camelot moment.

A Brush with History

On August 7, 1963, while completing an exchange transfusion on a jaundiced newborn in one of the two operating rooms, I became aware of activity in the adjoining suite.

After finishing the procedure, I pushed through the swinging door that connected the two rooms. A nurse was bustling about, making preparations for surgery. "An emergency C-section is coming in," she said, then added, "Why don't you hang around?" Within a minute or two, the main corridor doors opened, and on a gurney, guided by two corpsmen, lay Jacqueline Kennedy.

Devoid of make-up and pale in the harsh overhead light, her face betrayed little anxiety as she was transferred to the operating table. My perception of Mrs. Kennedy had been that of a delicately featured, fragile lady, more inclined to the salon than the playing fields and the strenuous pursuits of the Kennedy clan. Now, watching her, I was struck by the strong facial structure, broad shoulders, and sharply defined muscles of her upper arms. Certainly more the look of an athlete than I had suspected.

Most hospital personnel were aware of Mrs. Kennedy's pregnancy, of her due date in mid-September and her wish to stay on Cape Cod through as much of the summer as possible. Rooms had been prepared in the event she went into labor prior to her return to Washington. The choice of a military hospital, rather than civilian, presumably stemmed from her wish for privacy, which could be assured.

Her private obstetrician, Dr. John W. Walsh, arrived. After the two had a brief conversation, Mrs. Kennedy was prepped and medicated, and the surgery commenced. Present in the OR – other than the operating team – were myself and the two orderlies who had brought her to the surgical suite.

As he began the procedure, Dr. Walsh asked, "Who's here for the baby?"

The nurse assisting him nodded toward me and indicated I was on the pediatric service and available. He looked up briefly, then resumed his work.

No longer a spectator, I got myself ready. Within minutes, scrubbed and gloved, I was handed a tiny (4 pound 10.5 ounce) male newborn. Immediately it became apparent that the infant was distressed. The signs of inadequate oxygenation were obvious: rapid, shallow breathing, chest retractions, and bluish skin. After utilizing suction, postural drainage, and supplemental oxygen, we noted some improvement. The respirations, grunting to start, became less so, and then – most welcome – a short, shrill cry which repeated intermittently, initially with stimulation, but soon spontaneously. The infant's appearance, though hardly robust, had modestly improved as we prepared for transfer to the nursery.

The premature infant's respiratory difficulties presumed the diagnosis of hyaline membrane disease, now called infant respiratory distress syndrome. The condition is due to a lack of surfactant, a substance critical to lung expansion in the new-born. The treatment modalities in use today – CPAP (continuous positive airway pressure) and artificial surfactant – were not available until some years later.

As a result of this diagnosis being associated with the president's son, awareness of the disease increased, sparking further research. The odds of survival for an infant with a similar clinical scenario in 2015 are in the area of 95 percent.

The pediatric chief, Dr. Ed Jablonski, was waiting when we entered the nursery. As he conducted his examination of the baby, Dr. Stavig arrived with the president beside him. Ed offered his assessment of the infant's status and prognosis, which at that point was cautiously optimistic. When he felt it appropriate, the commander introduced those present to the president. In his accompanying remarks, Dr. Stavig mentioned my presence and assistance at the baby's birth. The president – tanned, shorter than I had thought, with a sun-induced auburn tint to his hair – shook my hand and thanked me, as he did all the others.

An attending physician at Boston Children's Hospital was en route to the Air Force base via helicopter. Soon after his arrival, the decision was made to transfer the baby to that facility. In spite of their ministrations, the infant's condition deteriorated, and in a last-ditch effort he was placed in a hyperbaric chamber, a treatment modality which provides oxygen under pressure to the lungs. The effort was unsuccessful. The baby, Patrick Bouvier Kennedy, died thirty-nine hours after his birth.

Several months later, on November 22, 1963, still attached to the pediatric service, I was working at a well-baby clinic. Suddenly, a loud radio disturbed the relative calm of the clinic. Annoyed, I went to the waiting room to ask that it be turned off. Shocked, I learned that President Kennedy had been shot and was reported dead. The assassination stunned and saddened the country, particularly our military community at Otis AFB, which the president had visited frequently en route to Hyannisport.

Meeting President Kennedy weeks earlier, albeit briefly, lent a poignant and personal dimension to the tragedy. My image of the president from that day – standing in profile beside the incubator, arms folded, one hand cupping his chin, his gaze focused on the frail wisp of humanity lying before him – has remained indelible.

Footnote: Patrick was buried in a family plot in Brookline, Massachusetts. In December 1963, he and his sister Arabella, a stillborn, were re-interred and placed alongside their father in Arlington National Cemetery.

On the Prowl

Cape Cod in summer, awash in pretty women, was the place to be for any single guy with a car and a couple of dollars in his pocket. Jack Chard, a flight surgeon, and I – two of the four physician bachelors on the hospital staff – shared these criteria.

Our goals relative to women were similar. There was occasional disagreement regarding pursuit tactics and capture management but otherwise we functioned well as a team.

Falmouth, Massachusetts, twenty minutes from the base, was our weekend launch pad. Preliminary visits were made to the various bars in town before we settled on the one with the best-looking women. The ladies, however, were not chosen willy-nilly. We had our standards: two arms, two legs, and most of their teeth. Sometimes – usually around closing time – these stipulations were substantially relaxed, deciding a winning smile really wasn't all that important.

If Falmouth became too crowded or manic, we repaired to Clauson's Inn just outside of town. Less frantic, and with dancing on weekends, it was close to the base in case any ladies wished to visit the officers' club for a drink and a dance.

The smaller crowd also better served Dr. Chard. Jack had poor vision but refused to wear glasses when pursuing women; he felt they detracted from the cool image he was trying to impart. His solution: on entering a bar, club, or lounge, he put on his glasses, scanned the crowd, and took a mental picture, then back they went into his pocket. A place like Clauson's, being less populated, worked to his advantage. (Jack, in fact, did have a photographic memory. A glance at a page for thirty seconds and it was his.)

His exchanges with women were imaginative. They began with the usual pleasantries, but eventually occupations entered the conversation.

"So what kind of work do you do, Jack?" a young lady would ask.

"Air Force," Jack might respond. As to what he did in the Air Force, Jack would lower his voice to a confidential level. "Test pilot." After a furtive glance over his shoulder, as though someone might be listening, he would add, "It's experimental, top secret. Can't talk much about it."

And on he'd spin, whispering of his supersonic adventures, never cracking a smile. A few of the ladies would catch on and think him and the story extremely funny, while others were true believers. Of the many occupations he trotted out on such occasions – CIA agent, Las Vegas lounge singer – the most successful was Hollywood talent scout ("looking for women for a new movie"). It was amazing how many ladies wanted to audition.

The major advantage Jack had over me when it came to attracting young ladies was in the automotive area. Jack drove an Avanti. I had a two-door 1955 De Soto. My vehicle wouldn't start unless a tongue depressor was placed in the air intake duct to keep the valve open, never an impressive start to a date unless she happened to be a mechanic. The passenger door, jammed and unable to be opened, was actually its best feature. The only available exit was on the other side of the driver, a delightful predicament and one that often took some time to resolve.

A Fortuitous Meeting

The 551st hospital was basically a long barrack with a series of wings extending from either side. At one end were add-on structures which housed the administrative and clerical section, offices for the commander, senior personnel, and the emergency room. Stretching in the opposite direction were two medical/ surgical wards, an obstetric unit which included the nursery, a six-bed pediatric unit, and a two-suite operating room unit.

Making rounds one Saturday morning during the spring of 1964, I eased myself into a crowded nurses' station to write orders and a progress note in a patient's chart. Present at the time was an unfamiliar blond nurse, the ward secretary, and an elderly female patient in a wheelchair enjoying a social visit. As I settled in at the small desk, the patient interrupted her conversation with the others to announce – in accented English – that "the doctor and the nurse would make beautiful babies." Never one to waste a line with such potential, I looked at my watch, then the nurse, and asked her how much time she had, which provoked a laugh.

The same nurse was at the officers' club that night, and although she didn't remember me from the morning – a blow to my ego – she did agree to a couple of dances. I learned her first name and that she was a member of a medical detachment from Boston, fulfilling their monthly active duty commitment. The exchanges both morning and evening were relatively brief, just long enough to fan a flicker of interest.

Flying School

Also, in the spring of 1964, the hospital commander called me to his office, an invitation fraught with negative possibilities: a patient complaint, a random chart review uncovering a discrepancy?

A smile accompanying Dr. Stavig's greeting eased my concerns. "An opening," he said, "will be available during the latter part of the year in the flight surgeon's office. I'd like to submit your name to headquarters for the position. Your decision is required in forty-eight hours.

When I mentioned the offer to Jack Chard, the flight surgeon for the fighter group on base, he said I should grab it. "Great bunch of docs in the office," he said "plenty of flying, chances to travel. Also the flight pay comes in handy."

I informed Dr. Stavig I was on board and looking forward to the assignment. Two weeks later I received official notification: the eight-week aviation medical program at Brooks AFB in San Antonio, Texas, was scheduled to begin in September.

The day before my departure, I purchased a sky-blue Ford Mustang from B.A. Dario in Pawtucket for $1,095 – my first new car. When I had asked my dad a few weeks earlier to join me on the trip, he jumped at the chance. The itinerary was loose with over-nights tentatively scheduled for Baltimore, Chattanooga, New Orleans, and Houston.

The trip began well but two personality traits – one his, one mine – became apparent, and if not resolved would have threatened the pleasure of our time together.

In my instance, I wanted to cover as much ground as possible each day which had us searching for places to stay well into the evening; for his part, he insisted that our accommodations be the least expensive of those available – even though it was my treat – which necessitated several stops until something finally met his frugal standards.

The situation came to a moderate boil in Chattanooga when I found myself at about 10:00 PM hung up in traffic searching for yet another establishment and a price comparison. We had been on the road about twelve hours, our respective moods reflected the weariness. A place presented itself, but the following morning I announced a plan to resolve the issue. Early starts in the morning were fine but at 4:00 PM or if we had traveled five hundred miles – whichever came first – we'd begin the search for a place to stay; he said that was okay and agreed the lodging could be my choice.

Holiday Inns made their appearance in the southern states – starting in the Memphis area – numerous enough to find one each night for the remainder of our trip. My father was delighted with the hotel, especially when I made up a number for the room charge substantially less than the actual price. We used the swimming pool, had a drink before dinner, and a relaxed evening. The new schedule improved the whole tone of the trip. We both looked forward to the next day's stop.

The World Series was in full swing, pitting the St. Louis Cardinals against the New York Yankees. Joe Garogiola was the play-by-play announcer. A former Cardinals catcher, he was a favorite of my dad, ever since he'd met him years before when Joe was playing for a local minor league team in Rhode Island.

Tooling through the countryside with his favorite (and only) son, the World Series on the radio, his "buddy" Joe announcing, my father was in his element, harboring hope all the while that the detested Yankees would lose. They did.

The only thing missing for him, the comfort that would have capped the experience, was a cigarette. A condition of the trip: no smoking. In retrospect, perhaps that was a mistake. In the fourth quarter of his pulmonary disease, the occasional cigarette would have given him something to look forward to a couple of times a day. Otherwise he had a great time and the Mustang, the coolest car on the road, performed admirably.

During the first weekend, we visited the Kennedy assassination site in Dallas, a few weeks shy of the first anniversary of the president's death. Guided tours of the San Antonio area filled my father's days; we hooked up for dinner in the evenings. He enjoyed the area, thought the people friendly, and "got a kick" out of the number of men – some on horses – who wore cowboy boots and ten-gallon hats. The Alamo, long on his wish list, was visited. Although he felt the drier air improved his breathing, strolls beyond a block were a painful slog. At the end of the week, he flew home. When we said our goodbyes he promised to add a daily prayer for success in my "flying" studies.

The class at Brooks was made up of approximately thirty physicians and twelve ancillary medical personnel. Most were military; the roll-call identified representation from USAF bases world-wide. The remainder worked in a civilian capacity; the FAA (Federal Aviation Agency) was well represented. A brief history of the flight surgeon inaugurated the program. During World War I the military hierarchy, dismayed by the high number of aircraft mishaps, commandeered a group of physicians to evaluate the air crews to ascertain if a physical reason could be contributing to the problem. The doctors found that a large proportion of the pilots had a variety of medical issues – vision being a primary offender – which should have been disqualifying at the outset. As a result, strict physical standards for fliers were enacted with a corresponding decrease in accidents. Thus was born the flight surgeon, the name something of a misnomer as very few are actually surgeons.

The primary focus of the course was to provide students with the information necessary to provide effective clinical care and support to flight-crew members. Over the eight weeks, that was accomplished with a variety of didactic and lab/technology presentations. Topics included aeromedical examination standards, medical issues related to flying, psychiatric concerns, in-flight medical emergencies, accident investigations, and hyperbaric medicine.

At many bases – including Otis AFB – occupational, preventative medicine, and military public health, came under the supervision of the flight surgeon's office. The course syllabus therefore involved: epidemiology, bio-statistics, toxicology, infection control, on-base civilian disaster programs, industrial injuries, and veterinary services, addressing our responsibilities in those areas. An intense program.

The only relief on the military side were the T-33 jet trainer rides out of nearby Kelly Field, though we never received any formal pilot training. One weekend I visited Del Rio, another brought me to Laredo (at that time a sleepy border town unaware of the mayhem soon to descend when the drug cartels set up shop).

My roommate, Rob, was a civilian physician who ran the Federal Aviation Agency (FAA) facility in Honolulu, and like myself, a country music fan. One Friday night we headed out of town, in the mood for a couple of beers and some good ol' country tunes. We were about thirty miles west of San Antonio driving in the general direction of Del Rio. Nothing had grabbed our interest, and it was getting late when we arrived at a deserted intersection. A right turn would keep us travelling west, a left headed us toward what appeared to be a small town off in the distance.

"What do you think, Rob?" I asked. "Right or left, you make the call."

"Why don't we give that place a shot," he said, pointing toward the collection of lights a few miles away.

As we approached, a billboard advertised a dance hall a half mile ahead which featured the great Bob Wells, considered the father of country music.

"I think we've found a home," Rob said smiling.

"Sounds good," I agreed.

Those were the days of George Jones, Roy Orbison, Ray Price, and Patsy Cline – the new kids on the block who replaced the likes of Lefty Frizell, Ernie Tubb, and Slim Whitman – when the look and sound of country music was changing. But the place that Rob and I came upon, a battered red barn with a bar and stage, was the real deal. An electric slide, two guitars, a fiddle, and banjo, along with a male and female vocalist, comprised the band. Anything beyond that – even piano – for folk in those parts was not country. The extravaganza of a Garth Brooks concert would have been beyond heresy.

Disparage if you will the hillbilly scene and its soppy music, but nights in that old hall, a couple of Lone Star beers aboard, the band easing into a country hurtin' song, and you've latched onto a tawny, tight-jeaned Texas cowgirl who dances like she means it, was not a bad way to spend an evening.

For his part, Rob - tall and gangly with an undisciplined thatch of reddish-blonde hair - preferred to hang out at the bar, sip his beer, listen to the music, and chat with the locals. A gimpy leg (sequela of a motorcycle accident) limited his dancing. Most of the men lining the counter and at the dozen or so tables, were in work clothes: battered cattle boots, denim shirts - some with vests - and worn jeans. All wore wide, soft-brimmed hats which were seldom removed.

Rob did become friendly with one woman, Laura, the manageress, who would – as befits a good hostess – chat and have the occasional beer with him. A tall, fine looking woman, she was always nicely sheathed in a form-fitting dress, a look quite distinct from the honky-tonk style – jeans, boots, and spangled blouses – of the other females. Her distinguishing feature: a wedge of white in her coal black hair at the center of her forehead.

Rob and I were there most Friday nights and the occasional Sunday afternoon. By the time our course at Brooks was finished, we were considered regulars and invited to come back anytime.

Our last night there – we were graduating in the morning – glasses were raised on multiple occasions to toast our good health and success. Laura must have arranged a night off, for she and Rob shared a table and drank some wine; she even got him on the floor for a couple of slow dances.

On the way back to the base I mentioned to Rob how lucky we had been to find the hall.

"Yeah," he replied. "I'm going to miss the place."

"After a while though," I added, "they all start to look the same. Like a rodeo, seen one, you've seen 'em all."

"Yeah, I suppose so," he answered, "but that one was a little special."

At the ceremony the following morning we were awarded certificates conferring flight surgeon status. After a few good-byes and an invitation from Rob to visit Honolulu, I fired up my Mustang and headed east.

Squadron Flight Surgeon

On my return to Otis AFB I was assigned to the 960th Airborne Early Warning (AEW) Squadron. Their aircraft – Lockheed EC-121 Constellations – flew triangular patterns along the northeast coast, their radar able to provide an early warning of hostile incursions. The Cold War era was at its height, and Russian aircraft were considered an existential threat to the major cities along the East Coast. The brinkmanship of the 1962 Cuban Missile Crisis was a recent memory. There were two other AEW squadrons attached to the base.

Also assigned to Otis was the F-101 fighter interceptor squadron. Their mission: confront, challenge, and contain any suspicious aircraft reported by the EC-121s. Two jets and their crews were on alert status at all times. The F-101 Voodoo was a two-man aircraft, with the pilot up front and the weapons control officer in the back seat.

A Strategic Air Command (SAC) group flying KC-97 aerial refueling tankers was also a tenant on base. They, too, were prepared, if word came down, to have a tanker airborne in a matter of minutes. During their seven-to ten-day rotations, the alert crew lived in a "mole hole," an underground living facility near the runway. The response aircraft was parked in close proximity. (This schedule raised havoc with the family situation; the divorce rate for SAC crews significantly exceeded that of other commands.)

Flight surgeons had a mandatory flying time requirement each month, thirty hours as I recollect. The rationale for this: the physician should maintain familiarity with the flight environment and working conditions of his patients. It could be satisfied with any of the flying units on base but the preponderance of hours was expected to be with your assigned squadron. Our primary medical responsibility was the health of the flight crews. An annual physical was conducted to include a comprehensive laboratory profile, chest x-rays, and an age-directed cardiogram. All squadron medical concerns were addressed by the assigned physician; a flight physician rotation handled issues after office-hours. This avoided the extended wait and occasional chaos of the regular emergency room and providers who may not have been aware of the treatment protocols for air crew members.

Their dependents were treated similarly to include routine pediatric and obstetric care; specialty referrals were arranged as necessary. Each of the five flight surgeons in the office were similarly trained and comfortable assuming these additional responsibilities.

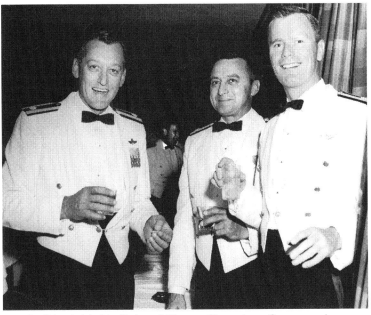

Left to right: Lt. Colonel Geyer, Squadron Commander;
unidentified pilot; and author

Although I had delivered the requisite number of babies during my residency, the training did not include the application of forceps, instruments used during the final stages of labor to expedite a delivery. Jack Chard, now my roommate, had more extensive OB experience and used them routinely. He offered me a tutorial.

One night over a beer, Jack gave his Forceps 101 presentation. At the outset he stated the reasons for considering their use and the reasons for not. More emphatically, he warned of the pitfalls that awaited if the procedure was done incorrectly.

"I only use Tucker outlet forceps," he said, "and take no chances. Only put them on when the baby's crowning, the scalp showing about the size of a fifty-cent piece. If the mother's exhausted, just can't push anymore, and the baby's right there, it's great to be able to give her some help." He laughed. "You want to see a grateful mama?"

"How about anesthesia?" I asked.

"Saddle block. Just like a spinal tap, except you inject lidocaine. Numbs her almost to the umbilicus. Get the episiotomy done, and you're ready to go. With the anesthetic aboard you're committed to forceps. That's the only way that kid's going to get delivered. So you gotta be sure they're on right."

One afternoon Jack borrowed a pair of forceps from the obstetric unit and purchased a melon – the approximate size of an infant's head – both of which he brought back to the BOQ. Although not the ideal method of instruction, it was enough to illustrate what the forceps looked like when properly placed and the technique used to get them there. After multiple applications over the next couple of days – same melon – I felt ready for the real thing.

I attended Jack's next two deliveries, and with patient permission, applied forceps and delivered the babies without mishap. Another two deliveries were accomplished in a similar manner with Dr. Cobb, the OB chief. With his blessing, I used my newly acquired skill on multiple births during the remainder of my Air Force career.

A Flight of Fancy

Over a drink at the officers' club bar one night, a SAC pilot mentioned an upcoming flight to Berlin. If I hadn't been there before, he said, I should come along. Never had I set foot in Germany, but I had visited many times, at least twice with John Wayne, once with Lee Marvin, and with other assorted movie actors. I'd flown its skies, roamed its fields, and romanced its women. So I knew Germany quite well. But in case I had missed anything, I told my pilot friend I'd be delighted to join the crew.

The aircraft was a KC-97, SAC's "aerial gas station." The flight plan took us to a mid-Atlantic rendezvous with two F-100 fighter jets which we'd refuel, then on to Keflavik, Iceland, to top off our own tanks. After an overnight in England, we'd fly on to Berlin.

Refueling procedures have their share of angst, especially when weather conditions are poor and the recipient of the exchange doesn't have an awful lot of time on his side. One of the challenges faced: slowing the jet's speed – already on the edge of stall – to that of the propeller-driven tanker. Often, to increase its speed, the KC-97 was put into a shallow dive. This was the procedure used the day I observed my first aerial refueling.

Standing behind the boom operator – the gentleman who manages the fuel transfer – the views were spectacular as we started the descent from our 32,000-foot cruising altitude: the broad, gray ocean below; the limitless sky above; the F-100 pilot clearly visible about twenty feet away. Given a head-set, I was able to hear the chatter between the aircraft.

The boom – a rigid, telescoping tube containing the fuel line – was released.

The pilot popped the cover of the fuel port, and the trick now was to hook one up with the other. Moderate to severe turbulence added to the difficulty. On the first attempt, the hydraulically operated boom was within inches of the hook-up when a run of bumpy air pushed the jet beneath us – and out of range.

The boom operator, Sgt. Ted, hunched over his instrument panel working the controls, urged the pilot on. "C'mon Sir, we can do this."

"I'm trying, Boomer," he replied. "Air's pretty rough."

The back of Ted's flight suit was stained with sweat. On the third try, the fuel nozzle had made it into the jet's fuel port, but the light on the control panel indicated it wasn't locked in and we disengaged.

Unfamiliar with the re-fueling procedure, I wasn't sure if what we were going through was standard stuff. But as turbulence bounced us around the sky, the planes advancing and retreating in a high-altitude *pas-de-deux* (at times a few feet removed from each other), it seemed a pretty dicey operation. My hands were wet, slipping on whatever I could grab to stay upright. A tightness had gathered at the back of my neck.

The second F-100 pilot, trailing in the distance, called in. "Getting pretty thirsty back here, folks." He mentioned the pounds of fuel he had remaining.

"You're next, Sir," Ted replied. "Haven't forgotten you."

You could hear his chuckle. "That's nice to know."

Our aircraft commander, a Lt. Colonel, called on the intercom, "What in the hell are you doing back there, Ted?"

"Getting it done, Sir. Moving right along."

"Hope so," the Colonel replied, "just went through twenty thousand."

"Yes Sir, I know."

Although the face of the F-100 pilot directly behind us was obscured by an oxygen mask and helmet, you could sense the tension building, hear the frustration in his voice, as the attempts continued. Finally, as we passed through 18,000 feet, he let out a whoop of relief when the coupling was accomplished and fuel flowed in his direction. The exchange completed, the pilot gave a quick thumbs-up and peeled off, a swoop of silver which seconds later was lost in the blue.

"A tough one," said Ted.

The second jet quickly moved into position. We were through the bad weather, the air smoother. His hook-up was accomplished on the first try. After a wing waggle and a "Thanks, Boomer," he, too, was on his way *That's when these hotshots really earn their money,* I thought. Just south of 10,000 feet we leveled off and began the climb to our initial altitude.

I talked to Ted later. He said they rarely attempt a re-fueling in turbulent conditions. They wait until they get through it or vector around it. "But these guys were on fumes," he said. "Had to take the chance."

The stop at the Air Force base in Iceland was brief: a fuel fill-up, a restock of food, water, and coffee, and we were airborne again.

We landed at the Royal Air Force (RAF) base at Mildenhall, which had achieved fame during World War II (even of the cinematic variety), for its role in the storied Battle of Britain days. Most bomber command missions to Germany originated there. Wellington and Lancaster bombers, soon joined by the redoubtable American B-17, leveled swathes of industrial Germany. The Spitfire and those who flew them out of Biggin Hill, Croydon, and the other fighter bases, made the headlines, but the unwieldy workhorses stationed here first brought the war to the Germans.

After a shower and meal, I wandered about the base looking for vestiges of its past. Little remained beyond the main building, which served as the command and operations center during the war. Runways had been lengthened, but there were no signs of commercial or military traffic.

In fact, the scene had the bucolic look of a Turner landscape. Scarcely removed from the runway were dense groves of trees, a field with cows grazing, smoke rising from chimneys in a nearby village, children laughing, and a group of boys playing soccer. A tableau which could have looked quite different were it not for the planes that had rumbled down these runways twenty-odd years ago when Hitler was at their doorstep.

Templehof Airport, where we landed after a three-hour flight from Mildenhall, was one of Europe's iconic airports in its day. The original construction in the mid-1920s had been upgraded during the Nazi era, with the hope of making Templehof the aviation centerpiece of the new Germany. The Allied victory altered that expectation; all flying activity, including commercial, ceased at the aerodrome in 1945. A brief resurrection occurred during the Berlin Airlift in the late '40s, when American C-54s and British transport aircraft used the airfield to bring food and fuel to Berliners.

When Germany joined NATO in 1955, the Luftwaffe was reactivated, with Templehof the home base for one of their interceptor squadrons. During our landing, a line of F-104s with German markings could be seen lining the tarmac. Also noticed were a couple of the grass/dirt runways used until the Berlin Airlift, when the heavily loaded aircraft tore the turf into massive divots, making safe landings unpredictable. Concrete runways were installed in a matter of days.

Our crew was put up in military housing at the periphery of the airfield. During the course of our chat with the building receptionist, an older German civilian, we wondered if there was anywhere we could get a beer. In excellent English he replied, "You would be welcome at the officers' club." He gave us directions and went on to say, "It's about the only thing around here left of the war years. Used by the officers back then and still today."

The club was a large space in the basement of one of the older buildings, with air and daylight provided by a series of windows placed just beneath the ceiling. About a dozen tables were scattered around an uncarpeted floor. They had a waxy feel as though leaching decades of sweat and humidity. Ponderous slabs of darkly stained wood dominated the scene, from the beams that stretched across the ceiling to the wainscoted walls and massive curved bar. The place smelled of must, stale beer, and cigarettes.

Four men were seated at one of the tables. All wore flight suits with F-104 insignias displayed on each arm. They introduced themselves as German pilots who had just flown in from Frankfurt for a week of training with the local F-104 squadron. After a brief chat, they returned to their table and beer. In a corner of the room, a blond, older woman playing an upright piano provided background music and the occasional lyric. Next to her on a small table was a pack of cigarettes and a half-drunk cocktail.

Beer was served from a large keg fixed to the wall behind the bar. The steins were frosted, the beverage cold and good. The three others at my table: pilot, copilot, navigator, bantered back and forth recollecting their active-duty tours in Europe and the war stories that go along with such conversations. My contributions were minimal – frequent nods and the occasional question – but I was fine with that. What my companions didn't know was that I had left, moved away in time, for me it was 1943.

The transition wasn't difficult. There I was, drinking Lowen-brau in a room where, in fact, the old Luftwaffe had congregated. German was being spoken at the next table, and the pilots using their hands to illustrate flying maneuvers, quite easily became the Stuka and Messerschmitt pilots of my imagination. They looked the part – blond, blue-eyed, with sharply angled features, the Aryan breed Hitler fostered and Leni Riefenstahl, the Nazi propagandist, filmed. The scene recalled a war movie I had watched as a youngster, starring Trevor Howard. The only thing missing was an imperious officer, wearing an Iron Cross, barking at a subordinate and a docile, gnome-like waiter who turned out to be a British spy. Even the piano player, her voice aged by cigarettes and songs too often sung, began to look and sound like Marlene Dietrich.

And then she was.

Dietrich's breakout movie of the 1920s was *The Blue Angel.* Her role was that of Lola, a cynical, sexually brazen cabaret singer who attracted men "like moths to a flame" and destroyed them as readily. The film tells of such a humiliation. A song from the movie was associated with Marlene Dietrich for the rest of her entertainment career. As though reading my thoughts, the blond pianist suddenly, softly, began to sing the timeless lament of a woman with too many lovers and too little love:

> *Falling in love again*
> *Never wanted to*
> *What am I to do*
> *Can't help it*
>
> *Love's always been my game*
> *Play it how I may*
> *I was made that way*
> *Can't help it*
>
> *Men cluster to me*
> *Like moths around a flame*
> *And if their wings are burned*
> *I know I'm not to blame*

As she played through the verses, there was a wistfulness in her voice, a look of bemusement on her face. Perhaps she was recalling the thousands of nights that had passed since she'd first sung the song, before her looks faded and her voice became a coarse whisper. As did Marlene Dietrich who, well into the last chorus of her career, trotted out the ballad time and again, becoming for a few moments the Lola of her youth.

When she finished, I, with a bit of unsteadiness, made my way to the piano, thanked her, and put a few dollars next to her cigarettes on the table. She smiled. *"Danke schön."*

A half hour or so later, we packed it in and started to leave. When we reached the door, I turned and tried to take a snapshot of the place in my mind so as not to forget. The lady at the piano waved good-bye.

As we walked back to the barracks, the navigator made the comment that although the beer was good, they should tear the club down and replace it with something more up-to-date. I said nothing, but for someone who had seen too many war movies as a kid, it had been a perfect night.

Thirty-eight years later in 2003, I, along with 30,000 others, ran the Berlin marathon. After the race, many of us recovered on the wide swath of green fronting the glass-domed Reichstag, while guzzling complimentary beer. Perhaps the setting prompted the thought, but sitting there I decided to visit Templehof before I left Berlin; maybe the officers club was still there.

As I walked toward a taxi rank the following morning, I suddenly realized how absurd it was to have such a notion.

Of course it's gone; it was a relic that night in 1964. Why tarnish comfortable nostalgia with gruff reality, risking certain disappointment? The memory of the evening remains fresh, the snapshot has yet to fade: Marlene still sings her song, and the beer is cold and good. Leave it be.

And thus it has remained.

In-flight Entertainment

Another notable flight experience took place a couple of months later which again involved a KC-97 aircraft, a flight to Europe, and a coupling, though of another sort.

The flight was a routine training exercise which didn't involve a re-fueling component. Other than the flight crew, the passenger roster included a half dozen airmen, an attractive blonde nurse, Bonnie (who worked in obstetrics in our hospital at Otis), and me. We were on leave, hitching a ride to our eventual destination, London.

Well into the flight, the nurse went forward to the cockpit to chat with the pilots. (Perfectly appropriate and before the flight was finished the airmen had done the same.) But a short time later, she returned...not alone. With her was the co-pilot: tall and blonde; the bars on his shoulders indicated the rank of captain. Smiling as they passed, they walked to the cavernous rear section of the plane and disappeared from sight. *The mile-high club is alive and well,* I thought. *Still taking in new members.* The airmen exchanged knowing smiles.

The co-pilot seat now vacant, I went forward to claim it until he returned. Arriving in the cockpit I saw both seats were empty. Curled in the space below the flight controls was the pilot, a major, fast asleep. After the initial surge of panic, I eased into the right seat and considered my options: go to the back of the plane and pry apart the lovers, wake up the pilot, or do nothing. The plane, obviously on auto-pilot, was proceeding smoothly, and at the moment, not requiring attention. If anything changed, I reasoned, I'd wake him up. So I made a command decision – at this point I felt in command – and did nothing.

The cloudless, star-studded night was splayed out before me; the moon, a sliver away from full, lightened a broad reach of black ocean. Although nervous about the situation, the hypnotic drone of the engines allowed a calmness and with it a hint of the surreal. Thrust five miles into the sky, a speck of metal inching through its vastness, brought a sense of insignificance along with an eerie feeling of being completely alone in the universe –in spite of the body snoring softly on the cockpit floor.

The situation resolved about twenty minutes later, although it felt longer. The cackle of chatter on the radio roused the major. He unwound himself from the cramped position, said "hello," and resumed his seat. He didn't seem surprised to see me sitting there.

The co-pilot returned a few minutes later, a grin stretched across his face. He thanked me for keeping his "seat warm," put on his head-set, and we continued along as though nothing had happened. It was one of those situations which when recollected the following morning makes you wonder if it were all a dream.

But the show wasn't over. We had the landing coming up. As we began our descent, I returned to the cockpit. At that time, when an aircraft came into range of the destination airfield, a glide path was set up by air traffic control. A visual display appeared on the plane's instrument panel to lead the aircraft onto the runway.

During the final approach, the air traffic controller (ATC) monitored the plane's progress at intervals, informing the pilot of his position relative to the glide path. Our pilot, the major – an older man, gray-haired – would have none of that, deliberately flying well above or below the prescribed path.

"Twenty feet above glide, Sir, please correct," advised the ATC, followed a moment later by advice to climb.

The major continued to play the game, the controller increasingly frantic, his English accent slurred with agitation, the closer we got to the field.

"Right now, Sir, pull up, you're twenty-five low."

About a half mile from touchdown, the major, grinning away, adjusted to the proper angle and landed.

"Why do you do that, Sir?" asked the co-pilot.

"Just to bust their balls."

The co-pilot and Bonnie hooked up later in London; we had a three-day layover before heading back. They were an item for a while at Otis, but I don't know if the romance that began so notably, survived or faltered in its course.

An Unlucky Coin Toss

In early 1965, the hospital was tasked with providing a flight surgeon for temporary assignment to Vietnam. Jack Chard and I both wanted to go. The others in the aviation medicine group – all married – had not expressed an interest. Dr. Stavig indicated that between us we could make the decision; he just needed a body.

One night after a couple of beers, we had a two-out-of-three coin toss to decide our futures for the next six months. Jack won the toss, and within two weeks he was Vietnam bound.

We kept in touch. He reported that the assignment had him jockeying between a couple of installations in remote areas of the delta, reachable only by helicopter. His patient clientele included both Army and Air Force troops and civilian Vietnamese. The conditions in the jungle that our guys had to fight in, he said, were horrendous; he expressed real doubt that the American campaign was going to turn out well. Coming from someone so gung ho and positive about our role there, that was a rare admission. He did manage trips to Laos and Cambodia, and some great war stories were promised.

When Jack returned, his intuition that the war in Vietnam was probably unwinnable had hardened to belief. "We can bomb them until the cows come home," he said, "but you're never going to get them out. And you got our guys slogging through swamps in heat you can't imagine. The VC come out of nowhere, pick a few of them off, and slip back into the jungle.

"Medically, dehydration is the biggest problem. After a patrol they all come back dry. Hell, they can lose five pounds in a day. There was stuff I'd never seen before – snake bites, weeping sores that cover every inch of bare skin, feet green with fungus, skin sloughing off in their boots. Unbelievable stuff."

"So what's the answer?"

"There is no answer. We're fighting in their neighborhood. And there's way more of them than there are of us. They'll knock those poor bastards off one by one until no one is left."

Since I was living in base-housing, our contact was mostly limited to the hospital. His active duty commitment was completed within three months. Jack liked the military and had given considerable thought to making it a career. His attitude changed after Vietnam. He was affected by the experience, the movie not as good as the trailer.

A final bash at the officers' club with a few friends from his squadron, some of the docs, and a couple of nurses, and he was on his way.

Back to his California roots, Jack established a family practice in San Clemente, married, and had a flock of kids. We kept in touch for a few years, but gradually the intervals increased until contact ceased altogether.

Memories of Jack – from his unique sense of humor to his California cool – always conjure a smile. His professional skills and easy rapport with patients ensured a successful practice, and I'm sure he's become a respected and stalwart member of the community. Whatever his achievements or enhanced status may be, the Jack I'll recall was a good friend back in the day, when both of us were younger, our resumes thinner, when he was a "test pilot," and I drove a De Soto with benefits.

The Flying Life

As predicted, travel opportunities increased with membership in the flying community. The EC-121s participated in frequent cross-country training missions; a SAC KC-97 flew to Europe every ten days. During the first quarter of 1965, I was appointed chief of aerospace medicine at the hospital, which warranted commercial travel to regional and national meetings. My squadron flight time requirements were accrued in the EC-121s – long, boring, twelve-hour missions over the Atlantic.

The most exciting flying experiences were in the back seat of the F-101s. Mock dog fights were staged high above the White Mountains in New Hampshire; hostile interceptions simulated over the Atlantic. Losing power in an engine was an occasional occurrence; the Voodoo's second engine served as a comforting backup, especially in over-water situations. Survival time in the ocean was in the neighborhood of thirty minutes, even when wearing exposure gear.

On one sun-drenched morning with unlimited visibility and only a few puffs of cloud, I was in the back seat of an F-101.

The pilot – and wing commander – Colonel "Skeets" Gallagher asked, "Have you ever been through the sound barrier, Doc?"

"No, I haven't," I assured him.

"Shall we give it a shot?"

"Sure, why not?"

Boston control was contacted, open airspace identified, the flight plan accepted.

"You okay back there?" the colonel asked.

"Yes, Sir," I replied.

"Then let's do it."

The colonel banked east, climbed to 35,000 feet, and on clearing the coast, lit the Voodoo's afterburners; the force of the acceleration drove me back into the seat. As the velocity increased I loosely gripped the handles built into the arm rests (when squeezed, you ejected from the aircraft). Within a minute we were approaching 500 mph; the speed increased evenly until we hit the 660 mph mark, the speed of sound at that altitude. At that point the air speed indicator needle slowed then fluttered, as if we had come to a barrier, as sailors report when butting against the Gulf Stream. The colonel pushed the aircraft nose forward. Within seconds a jolt was felt; the plane buffeted briefly then the vibrations cleared. The needle on the speed gauge spun backwards and settled just beyond Mach 1. We were through. The sensation of speed was not apparent until we leveled off and encountered high-altitude clouds building over the ocean. We sliced through them as if shot from a gun.

"What do you think, Doc?" the pilot asked.

"A day to remember. Thanks, Sir." My flight gloves were stuck to my hands.

"You're welcome."

He throttled back, put the jet in a sweeping, G-heavy turn, and angled back to the coast. We were on the ground in twenty-five minutes. A wild ride.

Joining Forces

My connection with Pat, the nurse captain from the medical group out of Boston, whom I met during the summer of 1964, had been maintained in sporadic fashion. Through the spring and summer of 1965 our meetings became more frequent, and it became obvious that what we had going was more than a summer fling.

Then autumn came, a particularly splendid New England Indian summer. For us it was a special time: a stretch of uncluttered days; lazy lunches in musty taverns; holding hands on steamer decks; Nantucket, wild and blowing; and long walks on barren beaches. It was on such a walk on our favored Old Silver Beach, the day desolate and gray, that we made the decision to join forces. So it came to pass that Father Quinn, a military chaplain we had met at Otis joined us in matrimony on September 29, 1965, at Saint Rose's Church in Chelsea, Massachusetts.

Our plans were less than precise, no carefully considered blueprint had been drafted, the future measured in months, not years. But we felt some traits held in common boded well for success: the willingness to take a chance, good sense of humor, a capacity to work hard, and the belief that no matter how bad things were today, there's always tomorrow. Blessed with youth and good health we were ready to take on whatever the gods had prepared for us – and still are, some fifty years later.

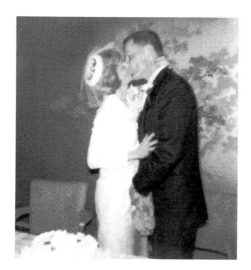

Wedding reception

DECISION TIME

M y USAF active duty commitment would conclude September of 1966. The decision about where to go from there loomed large on the horizon. The choice took on added relevance with the news that my blond nurse was dining for two.

There were options. The first and easiest: remain in the military and seamlessly retain the advantages of job security, advancement, worldwide assignments, and the host of benefits available to its members. I had been accepted at Ohio State's Aerospace Medicine Program which, if successfully completed, would provide a master's degree which would move me into the upper echelon of aviation medicine, with improved promotion potential and assignments.

Pat would have been quite content if we had remained in the service. Although I enjoyed my military experience, I felt that over the long haul I would chafe at the structured environment. There was also the sense that you lived at the mercy of an anonymous cipher in Washington, with little input as to where you would spend the next seventeen years of your life. Another element: the lack of challenge. If you turned up for work each day and kept your nose clean, you could cruise through your career. The job security of the military, in a perverse way, discouraged anything beyond a modicum of effort.

My thinking crystallized one day during a dental visit. Bibbed and waiting for the dentist to arrive, I noticed a calendar on the wall with X's marking the passage of days up to the present date. "What's with the crosses?" I asked the arriving dentist, an older, hump-shouldered lieutenant colonel.

"Marking the time till my retirement," he answered. "Counting the days to when I can finally get the hell out of here." He went to the sink, washed and dried his hands. "You know, Doc, I've been doing this shit for almost twenty years. Six months to go." His tone was less of anger or bitterness and more a statement of fact, like a prisoner about to be released from jail after serving his twenty-year sentence – not a heck of a lot to say, emotion having drained away years before.

"So," I asked, "why didn't you get out, go off on your own?"

He smiled. His teeth were nicotine stained. "For the worst reasons: security and the easy road. You and me, we're both in the same racket. You never have to worry about making a living or working too hard. I see a dozen or so patients a week, and that's it. A couple Scotches at night, a new X on the calendar in the morning. Just keep rolling along."

He turned off the overhead lamp, went to the room's only window, and looked out for a moment before turning back. "Twenty years of my goddamn life," he said, "and what have I got to show for it? Nothing, that's what, except a paid-off condo in Florida. On a golf course." He shook his head. "Should have taken the chance. I didn't know any better. But you know what the real kicker is?"

I shook my head no.

He smiled. "I don't play golf."

He switched the light back on, adjusted his face mask, took an instrument from the tray, and told me to open my mouth. At that moment I knew with certainty that I didn't want to be having a similar conversation in twenty years.

Another option: joining a private practice. Such an offer came from the physician father-in-law of a lady I had delivered. He was a Holy Cross graduate with a practice in Winchester, Massachusetts. Pat and I visited, and though impressed with the location and his flourishing practice, we decided against it. It looked too permanent. Neither of us, temperamentally, were ready to settle in for the long haul just yet.

At that time, the major airlines – Pan Am, TWA, United – were enjoying their glory days, bolstered by the advent of commercial jet travel, a public increasingly taking to the sky, and improved route structures and destinations. For obvious reasons, the carriers actively recruited well-trained military pilots who'd logged significant flight time and had experience flying multi-engine aircraft. The usual private pilot had yet to acquire such a resume. Not only were pilots actively sought, but also flight surgeons. The larger airlines had hubs scattered about the country where most of their workforce – both flight and ground – were located. As both a convenience and a cost-saving measure, it made sense to have physicians available to address medical concerns of these employees.

I discussed it with Pat, who agreed it might be an interesting transition before we settled into the cozy-cottage, white-picket-fence scene. Resumes were sent to three airlines, and two responded.

I interviewed in Kansas City with Dr. Charles Gullet, Trans World Airways (TWA) Medical Director, and in Chicago with Dr. George Kidera, United Airlines (UAL) Medical Chief. Within a week I received a job offer from each company. The open slot with United was at their flight training facility at Stapleton Field in Denver, while the TWA vacancy was in Los Angeles. As outlined by Dr. Kidera, I would be working with another physician presently in place, and we were expected to give talks (on medical issues related to flying), to newly-hired pilots, along with the usual medical tasks. That sounded interesting. The pay was comparable in both instances; the location and duties tilted the scale in favor of UAL. Pat was in agreement, so Denver it was.

Mile High Days

The housing concern was resolved through the intervention of Dr. Richard Harper, the physician working in the Colorado facility. A friend of his was offering a two-bedroom rental in Littleton, a suburb of Denver. He vouched for the neighborhood, the condition of the place, and its convenience to work. I rented it sight unseen.

Discharged from the military, I drove to Colorado with my father, leaving Pat and newborn Matthew in Massachusetts.

My dad, as always, didn't hesitate when asked if he were up for a trip. Comfortably ensconced in the passenger seat, he was content to watch the world pass by while following the journey on a road map, if in unfamiliar territory. For him, that included everywhere west of Chicago. We employed the same travel strategy that had worked so well on the Texas trip.

The last day of our journey began in Lincoln, Nebraska, and continued through the heartland of America, across the Great Plains. For mile after mile, reaching into early afternoon, we passed through vast stretches of grassland and wheat fields extending as far as the eye could see in every direction. It was a solitary drive only six or seven cars encountered the entire morning.

We stopped at a two-pump gas station, where a sign directed us to "the house on the left if you're looking at the station. Ring the bell and Jim will come out." Jim was the last person we saw for the next fifty miles. Inexplicably, when we did come to an intersection with another road, there was always a traffic light. Sitting there waiting for the light to change when we hadn't seen a vehicle for the past hour seemed bizarre.

In midafternoon the Rocky Mountains emerged in the distance, hazy at first, their large shadow grew more distinct until, by late afternoon, the snow-capped peaks loomed before us, silhouetted in the evening sky. Seeing how delighted my father was with our day of travel and "finally seeing the Rockies after all these years," made taking the job with United, however it turned out, worthwhile. This was my first time driving to Colorado, the only mode of travel, I believe, which allows the vastness of our country to be appreciated. Unfortunately, my father couldn't tolerate the thin air of the mile-high city. Unable to climb stairs and walk more than twenty-five feet without having to stop, and more significantly, awakening distressed during the night, he couldn't wait to board the first plane available to Boston. Within forty-eight hours he was airborne. It was an unfortunate ending to an otherwise very enjoyable trip.

Although I was on UAL's payroll and had already started work at their facility, retaining my position was contingent on passing the Colorado state medical license examination. Approximately two months after my arrival, I took the exam and passed, and with that pressure out of the way and an airline mechanics strike recently settled, Pat and Matt flew out to join me. Each morning I drove from our rental in Littleton to Stapleton Field and the United facility. In the distance, pocketed at the base of the Rockies, Denver was often wrapped in a mantle of smog. This problem was addressed by the city, and within a few years Denver had resolved the issue and now boasts one of the cleanest environments in the country.

My new son and I were getting acquainted. The day he was born I was taking the Massachusetts state licensing examination; I received the news during a lunch break phone call to the hospital. Until the exam re-start, I walked around Boston Commons trying to get my head around the fact I was a father *This is a whole new ballgame. A huge responsibility. Am I up to the task?* (Four children later the same question was being asked.)

Pat adapted quickly to her new role, and following in her wake I made reasonable progress. I learned quite rapidly that life would never be the same again. Every decision, every move, every aspect of my day would be considered in light of its impact on our new family member. The thought also occurred that the same efforts had been made for me at an earlier stage of my life, an involvement I more fully appreciated.

Matthew was a keeper from the start. Blonde, blue-eyed, a full-cheeked cherub with a goofy smile, he was his mother's "happy moment" – a title he carries to this day. His sunny disposition made things easy. As the weeks went by, my anxiety abated. I awarded myself a solid B in Fathering 101. (I chose not to seek anyone else's opinion.)

Dr. Harper and I got along well. A former Navy flight surgeon in his thirties, Dick was an easygoing guy with a great sense of humor. We alternated medical talks with the new hires and shared clinic responsibilities.

Three evenings a week I moonlighted at the outpatient psychiatric clinic at Denver General Hospital. My primary responsibility: updating patients' records with progress notes and refilling prescriptions.

The new-hire pilots were accepted into United's flight training program with the proviso that they pass the company's physical examination. Though they were a healthy group, the requirement nevertheless caused anxiety for some. Most were married, many with kids, and had already cut ties with their previous employers, predominantly military. They could ill afford to be rejected at this stage of the process. In very few professions does one's continued livelihood depend to such a degree upon the successful completion of the physical exam.

The more apprehensive of the candidates were easily identified: constant chatter, frequent questions, always in motion. Most settled down with casual conversation, peppered with reassurances. A small subset didn't. Moist skin, rapid pulse, and elevated systolic blood pressure were commonly present, and on some occasions, traces of sugar in the urine and electrocardiogram (EKG) changes. Any stimulus able to alter physical signs to the extent that organic disease is mimicked deserves serious consideration.

Propranolol (Inderal) had recently come on the market as a hypertension medication, its efficacy a result of blocking the effects of adrenergic (adrenaline) stimulation. An off-label use continues to be as a stage fright preventative. I wondered: what would happen if the adrenaline response to stress were blocked? With that stimulus neutralized, would the abnormal physical signs and EKG changes seen in the susceptible individuals no longer be evident? If so, you could conclude that the abnormalities were a result of stress, not disease. If, on the other hand, they didn't resolve, an organic cause would have to be considered. A handy method of differentiation it would seem.

An informal study was begun. Candidates who fit the anxiety/abnormal signs model were given a small dose of propranolol. Forty-five minutes later, the exam, lab, and EKG were repeated. In each instance, pulse and blood pressure became normal, and EKG and urine abnormalities, if previously present, were reversed. Subjectively, the candidates felt more relaxed.

The possibility of using the protocol as a routine with new hires that fit the profile was discussed with Dr. Kidera, UAL's medical director. Although he agreed with the concept and thought the results "interesting," he decided against its use system-wide. He felt the sample too small and doubted it would receive FAA approval. A more practical concern persisted: If this was the candidate's reaction to mild stress, did you want him flying your airplanes?

Aspen Airways

My introduction to skiing took place – as planned – during that winter. Aspen Airways provided service to the eponymous town. Nearby Vail was the new kid on the skiing resort block, having been incorporated just five years earlier.

The Aspen Airways fleet consisted of three refurbished, unpressurized military DC-6s. My first flight experience with them was the prototype for those that followed.

While waiting to board, I saw a large person wearing a cowboy hat lumber across the tarmac and climb into the plane. A moment later he reappeared in the cockpit and squeezed himself into the left seat; this was our captain. The copilot, as it turned out, was with another man, loading bags and skis into the rear of the aircraft. The precise weight of the luggage had been determined at the check-in counter. In the thin air, excess weight might, we were told, prevent the aircraft from lifting off the runway.

Once we were airborne, passengers were asked to remain in their seats until the flight's conclusion. "If two or three of you move to one side of the plane to check out the scenery," the copilot warned, "the weight could make the plane tilt. So stay put." At intervals he strolled down the narrow aisle with an oxygen canister for passengers who might be experiencing breathing difficulties. All the passengers – eight total–were told to check their fingernail beds frequently. A blue tinge was to be reported with a shout over the engine noise to the pilot in the right-hand seat.

Threading our way between massive, snow-capped peaks, riding the wind drafts sluicing through the narrow canyons, watching ice suddenly form on the wings and as quickly disappear, was not my usual flying experience. The views, however, were spectacular.

When we encountered heavy clouds about twenty minutes into the flight, the ground disappeared; we were flying blind. A couple of passengers expressed their concern, with the proximity of the surrounding mountains a recent memory. "No problem," replied the copilot. "We hook into a radio beam that takes us through a slot right into Aspen. When they hear us over the field, they let us know and we circle on in." And that's what they did. The DC-6 made a series of tight circles until the airstrip came into view, and then we made a routine landing. During the whole procedure the two pilots were chatting and sipping coffee. It was a walk in the park taken two or three times a day.

Weekends gave Pat and me the opportunity to explore the mountains, climb the continental divide, and visit old mining towns: Cripple Creek, Central City, and Leadville, where Oscar Wilde famously entertained the miners on his visit in 1882. United's flight perks allowed me on two occasions to bring my father and Pat, with her mother, on trips to Hawaii. They both enjoyed the first-class flying experience and the beauty of the islands that neither had seen before.

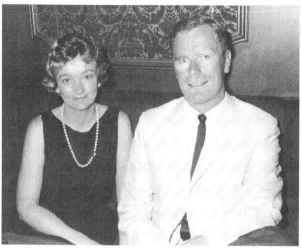

With Pat at Top of the Mark, San Francisco 1967

Colorado was a great experience for both of us, although Pat felt the isolation more than I, with a new baby and no car in a community that was a significant distance from the city. One weekend a month I was with the National Guard group at Lowery AFB. That, along with my psychiatric clinic involvement, didn't help matters. A miscarriage also occurred, which dampened the scene. So when an opening became available at United's facility at the National Airport in Washington, D.C., we decided to take the opportunity and move east.

A Capital Choice

Cherry blossoms were in bloom on the spring day in 1968 when we arrived in D.C. Our residence was a motel until a permanent situation could be found. United was quite helpful in this regard, making available a list of realtors who had done business with the company previously. Within two days we found a townhouse in Bedford Village, a recently completed complex in Fairfax, VA. Handy to the beltway – the major access to the District and shopping – it fit our needs perfectly.

Most of our neighbors, we soon learned, were in our age bracket, young married couples with small kids, many of the husbands working in the District for the government in either a military or civilian capacity. In a couple instances, friendships with neighbors became lifelong.

Dr. Bill Albers, a former Marine pilot, was the physician in charge of the UAL medical facility located in a hangar at the National Airport (since renamed for President Reagan). My responsibilities were similar to those in Denver but without the teaching piece.

My association with the National Guard continued as I attached myself to the hospital unit at Andrew's AFB in Virginia. I also found a moonlighting job: two six-hour shifts a week in the emergency room at Fort Belvoir, an Army base just over the Virginia border. One evening I shared a shift with Dr. Ned Healey, a classmate at Holy Cross.

We found Washington to be an exciting place: a cultural and intellectual oasis littered with artifacts of U.S. history and monuments to the founders at every turn. There was also a subliminal sense of being at the epicenter of power in the world. To Pat's relief, our social life improved. With friends made in Bedford Village, we enjoyed embassy parties, the Marine Corps Ball, Potomac cruises, a sampling of great restaurants, and house parties – a continuing succession of events that kept our calendar full. It was a far cry from the Denver days.

A strange experience enlivened an embassy tour one Saturday afternoon. Most of the embassies were located in the same area of the District, and several times a year the public was invited to view these very elaborate, well-appointed residences.

That afternoon, Pat and I were enjoying a tour of the Romanian embassy. I noticed a small, dark-haired man, a member of their staff, watching me. Each room we went into, he would look toward me for a moment, then walk away. I thought it strange and mentioned it to Pat who attributed it to my peculiar imagination.

The tour drew to a close; the little man reappeared. I was standing at the back of and a little apart from our group. Once again the stare but this time he approached, took a piece of paper from his pocket, handed it to me and scurried off. On the paper was a name, presumably his, a phone number, and in large print: "I want to defect to the USA." I showed it to Pat who couldn't stop laughing. The only words she was able to muster between bursts of merriment were, "my husband, the secret agent." As we left the building my new friend gave me a wave and a grin.

Imagining how John Le Carrè would handle the situation, I went to FBI headquarters. The agent, an older man with world-weary eyes and a cynical smile, wasn't too impressed. This happens frequently he told me, but "never Romania." In a cryptic aside he instructed, "Be available, McKee, in case the Agency needs your help." He paused. "We'll get the note upstairs to the Old Man, see what he wants to do." He took my contact information. We shook hands. His grasp was firm.

I don't know what happened to the man at the embassy, but in a strange way, I thought it quite a feather in my cap to be the one chosen from the group of visitors. Obviously he had seen in me the coolness and acumen required for such a clandestine operation. Our friends, hearing of my experience, referred to me (for a considerable time), as "secret agent." I took their barbs in stride, as you must when you're working with the Agency, determined not to let the episode affect my lifestyle or change my regular-guy image.

But I did buy a trench coat in case the FBI called.

A favorite Saturday excursion included lunch at O'Donnell's Seafood Grill on E Street. Their specialty: Maryland crabs with the succulent meat extracted, submerged in butter, cooked over an open flame, and served in small copper skillets with sweet buns for dipping. Preceded by a chilled, dry martini, the experience bordered on the sensuous. The remainder of the afternoon was spent browsing the myriad galleries and art exhibitions, with the Getty and Smithsonian museums repeat favorites.

Two significant acquisitions came about during our stay. One was short-term: the purchase – via the G.I. bill – of a house on Farmington Drive, a short distance from the town of Fairfax. The other was a lifetime acquisition: our daughter, Ellen, born at Fairfax Hospital on January 26, 1969 (also my father's birthday).

A retired cardiologist, Dr. John Smith, worked part-time with us at the UAL dispensary. We became friendly. I sat with him while he interpreted cardiograms, and with his tutelage over the course of months, I became reasonably proficient.

I talked with him about the study I'd done in Denver involving the anxious new hires and the results obtained when they were given small doses of the beta blocker. He considered it an interesting observation and thought others in the aviation medical field might find it useful.

"Write it up," he advised. "Present the clinical scenario, add some detail regarding the pharmacology of the drug and the physiology of the adrenal system, and discuss the clinical implications. Then get Kidera's approval and submit it to the *Journal of Aerospace Medicine*." With his help I did, and "Beta-adrenergic Blockade – An Aid to Diagnosis" was published in the *Journal* in June 1969.

Dr. Smith's interest was piqued to the extent that he did a follow-up article, properly controlled and with case studies, utilizing essentially the same protocol and achieving similar results. His piece, "Studies of the Effect of Beta-Adrenergic Blockade on R-ST Segment and T Wave Changes," was published in *Aerospace Medicine* in February 1970.

Dr. Smith had a cardiac condition, angina pectoris, or chest pain on exertion. He advocated exercise – specifically walking – as a treatment for the condition. Rather than halting the activity with the onset of chest discomfort, he advised patients to continue to walk, increasing the pace if possible, until the pain resolved. The exact mechanism that prompted the recovery was unclear. The abrupt and dramatic relief suggested a coronary vessel spasm suddenly released or, less likely, a collateral circulation that kicked in to supply the necessary oxygen.

Following his own dictum, John walked briskly twice a day. I occasionally accompanied him on his noontime foray around the National Airport parking lot.

It was quite a stroll. Five minutes into it, his pain began and remained as the activity continued. My suggestion of nitroglycerine – which he carried with him – was dismissed. He increased the pace. The discomfort was extreme, his face white and moist. Suddenly, the bolt of relief. "There it goes," he would say. Whatever the mechanism, blood now perfused his heart muscle. Dr. Smith, still maintaining his pace, was now smiling, face dry and a robust pink. "Greatest feeling in the world when it clicks in," he said. "You can't imagine." And he went through this routine twice a day!

As enjoyable as our stay was in the D.C./Virginia area, my feet remained itchy. There were also some issues developing with my colleague, Dr. Albers. My presence in the office had allowed him to slip into a semi-retirement mode. His frequent absences, arriving late in the office most days, strained our collegiality. But the greater issue: his insistence on total control. Routine lab work, physical exams, x-rays, and consultations, required his approval and co-signature. Stacks of physicals, various requisition forms and letters littered the office. Not a happy situation.

Over dinner one evening, I mentioned to Pat that there was an opening at JFK airport in New York. "What do you think?" I asked.

"We've just bought a house," she replied. "We're barely settled in."

"I know. So what do you think?"

"What about the friends we've made - the trips we had planned with them?"

We had become quite tight with two other couples whom we had met at Bedford Village. Most of our social outings included them. But they, too, I pointed out, were making plans to leave the area – one because of an upcoming military transfer, and the other, needing space for a growing family, was looking at homes in Maryland.

"Where would we live?"

Aha, she might go for it. "Probably on Long Island. Supposed to be nice out there."

"What about Georgetown?"

Serious consideration had been given to my attending law school there, with the thought of working in the medical/legal arena. The lawyer in my Guard unit at Andrews AFB was on the faculty at Georgetown. He was quite certain he could arrange my admission if I agreed to a military commitment upon finishing the program.

"It would be school full time," I said. "What are we going to live on, the four of us? That check every two weeks keeps it going for us. And it would be at least two years in school."

"Will United move us?"

"Yes, they'll put me up in a motel near the airport. I'll fly home on weekends. When I find a place to live, they'll pack us up and move us. Really not much for you to do, just point to what you want packed."

"How about this place? We've got a mortgage."

"United will take over the mortgage. We won't be stuck with it. They'll probably list it for sale with a local realty." I paused. Matthew, playing nearby, watched us with apparent interest. "Looks like he's in. What do you say?"

Pat managed a smile. "Do you think we can stay there a while?" Her voice wasn't dripping with sarcasm, more a subtle ooze.

"Absolutely," I replied.

An observation must be made. A limited cohort of women are able, at a moment's notice, to uproot themselves from the comfort of their homes, the company of good friends, and the security of familiar surroundings, and head (with kids) into the unknown. Some even give the impression of looking forward to the adventure, the excitement of something new. These women are found most consistently in the armed services, where frequent assignments come with the territory. Usually their husbands are career military. Those who couldn't adapt to the peripatetic lifestyle wouldn't still be around. Pat, it must be said, had something of the gypsy in her blood and was quite willing to give most propositions a shot. Which was appreciated by her husband.

On the Road Again

We purchased a house in Massepequa, on Long Island, and moved into it in May, 1969. George Catlett, MD, was in charge of the UAL medical facility at JFK. At that time George was a rising star in the Aerospace Medical Society hierarchy, having held positions of influence in that group for years. Elections were coming up, and I believe he was vying for its presidency. Much of his time was spent dealing with the political machinations required when pursuing such a goal. He gladly relinquished many responsibilities in the clinic to me.

From a medical perspective, the job – similar to others with United – wasn't challenging. Air crew populations rank among the healthiest in the nation, and their annual evaluations were, in most instances, confirmations of their good fortune. The injuries and occasional illness suffered by ground employees were usually not significant. Any malady of importance for either group would prompt a visit to their own physician; the less the company doctor knew of health issues which could impact their employment, the better. One thing I can say without fear of rebuttal, and I'm confident enough to risk money if any physician were to challenge me: when my waiting room at JFK was stacked with stewardesses (female flight attendants in today's vernacular), perhaps there for a physical, immunizations, or a medical clearance to return to flying, I had, hands down, the most attractive waiting room in America.

As had been my habit in other locations, I sought a moonlighting job. A surgeon that Dr. Catlett frequently used as a consultant, who lived on Long Island, suggested a friend of his with a family practice in Farmingdale. In something of an extraordinary coincidence, Dr. Bill Squires had been stationed with me at the 551st Hospital at Otis Air Force Base. I didn't know him well, but remembered him as having a savvy business sense. While at Otis, he worked nights and weekends for a physician in a medical group in Sharon, MA. Bill had organized a pool of physicians from the base to provide similar services for others in the group. He had the physical appearance and the aggressive charm of a Rod Steiger, as well as a reputation for being an excellent physician.

We met, and he expressed a willingness to establish some evening hours, both as a convenience for his patients and to decrease his daytime patient volume. I worked 6:00 to 9:00 p.m. three evenings a week. As it turned out, I couldn't have chosen a better apprenticeship for my eventual move to private practice.

Dr. Squire's practice included a full spectrum of diagnostic modalities: EKG, PFT (pulmonary function test), tonometry, audiometry (a handheld device), sigmoidoscopy, X-ray, basic blood profiles, urine culture and sensitivity, scratch testing for allergies, and basic orthopedics; he also offered diet and exercise programs and dispensed medications.

Apart from the medical experience, he provided an excellent introduction into the business aspects of a practice. For the first time since my Air Force days, I was enjoying the clinical side of medicine. The thought of getting back into family practice gained traction.

Soon after our arrival on Long Island, Pat experienced GI symptoms strikingly similar to those which had announced her previous states of being with child. After a tedious pregnancy and difficult delivery, our second daughter, Kathleen Ann, was born on January 16, 1970, at Bayside Hospital in Oyster Bay. She was one beautiful baby.

A Soft Sell

The conversation with Pat about two months later began with my comment about an approaching snowstorm and her adding, "It's been a miserable winter. I can't wait for spring, just to get the cold out of my bones." She was cradling a hot chocolate in her hands. Katy had just been fed, Ellen was asleep upstairs, Matt played contentedly on the floor. The frustration in Pat's voice was obvious. An arduous pregnancy had recently ended with little help from me, family, or friends. The social connections we'd enjoyed in Virginia were not replayed here. I was on the freeway by 7:00 each morning, returning around 9:30 three nights a week, with a National Guard obligation one weekend a month. Being home alone with three kids – one brand new – can get old after a while, especially when there is nothing on the horizon to brighten the picture.

"You know," I said, "we haven't been on a beach or in the ocean for two summers. Can't count that day at Jones beach. Even the water was crowded. Looked like the Ganges on a Hindu holy day."

My attempt at humor produced a shrug of her shoulders, a wan smile, and an unenthusiastic, "Maybe next summer."

While a gray fog stole what remained of the afternoon light, we talked about kids' issues, the upcoming visit of her mother, and possibly hooking up with a pharmaceutical company-sponsored junket to Barbados (which we enjoyed). As we chatted, the thought that had been nagging for a couple of months recurred: *Is now the time to bring it up – leaving the airline and going into private practice?* In my own mind the decision had been made. I wanted to do it. But with a new baby and two moves within two years, I didn't know how the idea would resonate with Pat. I did know she was not enamored of Long Island.

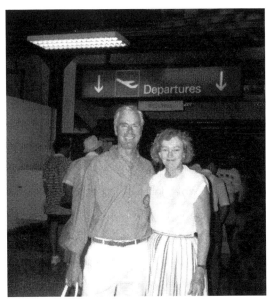
With Pat en route to Barbados

I had discussed my plan with Bill Squires, who thought it a great plan, with a "Why don't you come in with me?" addendum. But our practice styles and personalities were very different. This wasn't a problem in our present setup, but there was bound to be conflict if we worked together. I thought it best not to disrupt our friendship.

I briefly considered opening a practice on Long Island. However, the increasingly crowded suburbs and their loud, pushy populace, whom I battled with each morning on the freeway, as Pat did in the markets, was not the neighborhood either of us wanted for the long term. Whatever decision we reached, I had decided to leave United. Though a good company with great perks, the duties of the physician in their medical departments were repetitive (endless physical exams), offered few challenges, and didn't provide the personal satisfaction found in dealing with sick people, especially if they got better.

The three years were a remarkable experience for Pat and me: our assignments, friendships made, travel that took us from the majestic Rockies to the swaying palms and fragrance-laden breezes of Hawaii. It had served its intended purpose as a transition from a period of uncertain career intentions to one where the path was more certain. Now was the time to make the move. Sometimes you just know.

These thoughts percolated in my brain that winter day as we chatted. *At least throw the idea out there*, I prodded myself. *Get the conversation started.* Pat was talking about a well-baby appointment the following week when I interrupted her.

"Pat, I've been thinking about something for a while."

"Really?" she replied. "What about?"

"Leaving United and going into practice on my own."

"Is this a joke?"

"No, dead serious. You're not crazy about this place. Why don't we get the hell out of here and head home, back to New England?" Pat's family lived in the Boston area, and I knew she'd like to be closer to them.

She didn't answer. After a moment she set her mug on the adjoining table and drew her legs up beneath her.

Maybe a hint of interest.

"Where in New England?" she asked.

"Well, anywhere you like," I said, speaking quickly, "but I was thinking of Rhode Island. You'd love it there. Never far from the ocean. About a half hour from Boston. Plus, I have a Rhode Island license."

Ellen was fussing upstairs. I brought her down, and she cuddled next to her mother. Wind rattled the outside shutters, rain pelted the windows. I walked around the house and switched on lights but didn't sit down.

"Anyway, the move thing I was talking about," I said, my tone dismissive, "it was just a thought. No big deal. Probably shouldn't have bothered you with it." Mumbling something about a football game, I went into the den and turned on the TV. A strategic move. Would she or would she not follow me in?

She did, with Ellen in tow. "So this move," she began, "when were you thinking? A year or two?"

"No, now. As soon as I could find a place for us to live." I turned and faced her. "Shall I start looking?"

"We've got a lot to talk about still. Hmm...yes, I think I would like that." She paused. "But wherever is next I want to stay there a while."

"And you will."

Taking the Plunge

McKesson/Robbins, a major pharmaceutical company, distributed a free monthly newsletter similar to the classified section in a newspaper. It listed physicians seeking practice opportunities and vice versa, locum tenens offerings, practices for sale, doctors looking for assistants, and related information. I placed an ad indicating my specialty and my interest in joining a practice in Rhode Island.

Three weeks later I received a letter from Dr. Ernesto D'Agostino at South County Hospital (SCH), located in Wakefield, Rhode Island. A surgeon, Dr. Bob Conrad, had seen my ad and asked Dr. D'Agostino, then secretary of the medical staff, to contact me. His letter briefly described the hospital, the growing population in that part of the state, and the need for primary care physicians. He said he would be glad to meet whenever I was in the area.

Pat and I arranged a visit. The hospital was, as I remembered, a two-story brick structure astride an elevated stretch of land overlooking the Salt Pond. Dr. D'Agostino brought us through the facility, a brief meeting was had with the CEO, then coffee with two physicians. Later on we met with a real estate agent, Ken Munro, who agreed to handle the house search; contact information was obtained for the owner of a medical office building. The population of South County was about 18,000, Narragansett 7,500 with a 10 to 15% boost in the summertime.

After a late lunch at the Larchwood Inn in Wakefield, we drove around the area, which was familiar territory to me after a number of childhood summers spent in nearby Narragansett.

I selected a route which I hoped would display the community in its most attractive light.

The gods were with us. On this March day, Mother Nature was feeling it, strutting her stuff: briskness in the air but a warming sun, not a cloud in an azure sky. The fishing port of Galilee, with Jerusalem on the opposite side of the channel, was a postcard scene: trawlers in line, nets hung from their masts streaming in the breeze, seagulls squawking and wheeling around an incoming boat, the taste of salt in the air.

We followed a line of beach which, during the 1938 hurricane, was swept clean of hundreds of small, fragile cottages. A few new homes had been built along the still-desolate stretch, but the memory of the disaster was too fresh for many to tempt fate again.

"Is that smudge of land, out in the bay, Block Island?" Pat asked.

"Yes," I said. I mentioned a tale from my fish-cutting days. "Back in the early days of World War II, when Germany controlled the Atlantic, crew were known to have gone ashore there to pick up supplies. The story goes that their shopping also included a couple of the local ladies."

"I'm not too surprised," she replied, "German men are considered a pretty handsome bunch."

"I've got some Kraut blood in me, by the way. Just so you know," I said.

Pat turned and patted my shoulder, "then there are the exceptions."

Passing a scattering of Gatsby-like mansions and a string of weathered, gray-shingled homes, we came into the town of Narragansett. I pointed out the outlines of Jamestown and Newport, distinct on this low-humidity day. Just beyond an imposing stone archway, which I explained was the most visible remnant of the town's Roaring Twenties interlude, we parked and admired a splendid sweep of coast.

The placid bay was free of traffic, except for a large sail-boat motoring out of Newport. Before us, a ribbon of surf lined a broad, curved beach joined at its far end by a collection of dunes. Two fishermen were casting lines into the calm water. Just ahead, along the sea wall, a man in a wheelchair stared intently at the ocean, while his disinterested, young, male companion smoked a cigarette and frequently checked his watch.

"That old guy is looking at the ocean like he's never going to see it again."

Pat nodded, "Maybe he never will. But if this is his last look, he picked a beautiful day. And so peaceful."

"Glad you came?"

She smiled. "Maybe starting to grow on me a little. We'll see."

I didn't press it, but I knew she was hooked.

Over the next six weeks, plans inched ahead. A major difference between this move and the previous ones was, because I left United of my own volition, the task of selling our house and contracting with a mover fell to us. Getting the house ready to be shown to prospective buyers, often on short notice, created its own stresses, which fell primarily on Pat's shoulders. Luckily, a buyer was quickly found, and with that out of the way, a more certain schedule could be arranged.

My application at the hospital was accepted, a meeting with the board of trustees went well, and the new home and office space issues were resolved. Thanks to a wonderful older lady who took over the babysitting chores for all but the newborn Kate, the three of us took a trip to Claflins, a medical supply house in Quincy, Massachusetts. There, with the help of the State Street Bank, I arranged the purchase of furnishings and equipment for the office. By the middle of May, we were ready to make the move. Ten days later, family, luggage, and plants were packed into our Nash Rambler, and we headed north.

- PART TWO -

Practice Time

D r. D'Agostino held a reception at his home welcoming Pat, me, and another new arrival, Dr. Richard Judkins, a board-certified ENT physician. Most of the medical staff attended, able to fit comfortably into the living room of the home – an indication of the size of the staff at the time. Everyone was very friendly; all wished us well and offered their assistance.

A contract had been signed to rent office space, beginning June 1, at a medical building located in Narragansett. An announcement of my practice location and start date was placed in the June 4, 1970 edition of the *Narragansett Times*.

Arrangements were made for the office phone to ring at home. The plan was to work by myself in the office for the first few days – presumed to be less than busy – until babysitting had been arranged. Pat would then function as receptionist, secretary, and nurse, until those slots were filled. A major decision was made: the charge for an office visit would be $12 rather than the prevailing $10.

My first day in practice I saw ten patients, half of whom left with a scheduled return visit. They all paid me – most did in those days – so I made $120. I thought it a good start.

At about the two-week mark I hired a secretary, an older lady whom I'll call Elsie. Her resume included fulfilling similar duties for two other physicians in town. The one doctor I called heartily endorsed her. With that recommendation in hand, I didn't bother checking with the second physician. Her hiring freed Pat of her secretarial role, but still, babysitter dependent, she filled the other roles for months.

In order to stimulate business, I visited every physician in town, both as a courtesy and to offer my services on the days they were designated to cover the emergency room (ER) in the hospital.

A formal ER physician call schedule had only recently been put in place. Prior to that, a patient seeking treatment came to the back of the hospital. There, above a door, a sign indicated "Emergency Room." An arrow directed the caller to a red-colored doorbell which summoned a nurse. She appraised the situation and either treated the patient herself or called their physician for further instructions. Increasing volume necessitated a nurse being assigned full time to the small, windowless ER space in the basement.

Since trying to find the patient's doctor was often a tedious and unsuccessful exercise, a formal physician rotation was created. The on-call doctor did not have to be physically in the facility but prepared to come to the hospital if the nurse felt his intervention necessary. Most of the doctors I visited were delighted to have someone cover their rotation, and my offers were gratefully accepted. A full-time ER doctor was brought in during the late 1970s.

The practice, in its sixth month, was building nicely. Elsie was working out well, hours were expanding, and my volume was in the range of fifteen to twenty patients per day.

Two mornings a week I worked in Health Services at the University of Rhode Island (URI); this affiliation provided income for countless physicians new to the area as they established their practices.

The medical director at the time was Dr. Martin O'Brien. In his early seventies and Harvard-trained, he had, for many years, a private practice in Wickford. Formal in manner and professionally attired (starched white coat, cuff-linked shirt, tie and vest), he exuded the look of the patrician. Behind clear, rimless glasses, however, pale blue eyes glinted with humor. That attribute, I came to learn, best defined the man.

My interview with him during the hiring process went well. Our discussion covered what to expect when dealing with a younger population, dispensary resources, and my role. When I asked him if there was anything I should be aware of clinically, conditions in the collegiate setting which might not be encountered in my Narragansett office, his answer was concise. "You'll see more sex disease here than if your practice was in a whorehouse."

Profound societal changes initiated in the United States during the 1960s, blossomed the following decade – the transition illustrated most dramatically by shifts in sexual attitude and behavior. The "revolution" which promoted sex outside the boundaries of heterosexual marriage became more socially acceptable. No demographic welcomed this new-found freedom more enthusiastically than the college population. The key was the availability of birth control pills. Dr. O'Brien felt that 75% of female students were on some form of pregnancy prevention.

"This place is a regular rabbit farm," he said. "They're at it all the time." He shook his head, the look on his face a cross between amusement and amazement. "And then they come here for us to clean up the mess they made."

This I found to be true. More patients presented with concerns or symptoms related to their sexual activities during a week than I would see in a year of my practice. Gonorrhea (GC) was frequently encountered, the diagnosis in males obvious a few days after exposure: a penile discharge copious enough to stain underwear. But since symptoms of GC in females could be mild enough to go unnoticed, Dr. O'Brien had set up a protocol. Any sexual exposure with or without suspicious symptoms mandated a cervical swab, and dependent on history, cultures obtained from other body orifices. Dr. O'Brien described this activity as "looking for pecker tracks."

In his undergraduate years, Dr. O'Brien had minored in philosophy, an interest he informally maintained. That background influenced his thinking, and phrases such as, "existential crisis," "didactic implications," etc., peppered his conversations. He disagreed with birth control, not for moral or religious reasons, but because he felt it a disruption of the courting timetable, a period during which minds and personalities – not bodies – met, meshed, and became compatible – or not. He insisted this was the important component – the part you had to get right – of any relationship, "not the screwing." The good doctor never forced his thinking on to the students. He recognized battles he could not win.

Although blessed with a good sense of Irish humor, his choice of jokes was juvenile and beyond corny. "What's the mathematician's favorite dessert?" he would ask. Then, face flushed with mirth, came the answer: "Pi." A frequent greeting in the morning: "Gnid morning, Doctor." This made reference to gram negative intracellular diplococci, the GC bacterium. Dr. O'Brien felt this was hilarious.

My practice grew, and I discontinued my affiliation with URI Health Services. However, I remained in contact with Dr. O'Brien. Shortly after his retirement, I arranged – as president of the medical staff at the time – a farewell dinner for him at the Dunes Club. Many of the physicians who worked with the doctor at URI attended. I was able to find two members of his Harvard Medical School class who lived just over the Massachusetts border; they brought pictures and a collection of reminiscences. After moving through the complimentary and laudatory portions of the program, the evening evolved into something of a roast, with the good doctor returning (with equivalent deftness), the jibes received. The evening finished with his emotional farewell.

Occasionally passing through Wickford, I would see Dr. O'Brien, astride a sturdy, three-wheeled bike, its wicker basket filled with groceries. Our short conversation affirmed that things were going well.

"My major activity these days," he said, "is peddling my ass around town."

Much busier, I felt it was time to take on a full-time nurse. An advertisement was placed in the *Narragansett Times*, which yielded six replies. Within three weeks the position was filled.

The terms of employment: $7.50/hour, 35-hour workweek (variable), one week of vacation and a provision for sick time, no smoking in office. Nurses were expected to wear white (including shoes), and their nurse's cap.

The uniform stipulation did not, in 1970, provoke the dismay it might today. This attire was standard for nurses of that era, especially in the hospital setting. Their professional image was, in my mind, epitomized by the nurse's cap, a symbol as indicative of competence and authority as the Green Beret's head gear, the aviator's wings, or the policeman's badge. Remove the symbols and you've lost your identity.

Surveys have shown that patients equate the appearance of the nurse – and doctor – with the quality of care they receive. The sloppy, unkempt physician or nurse may imply a similarly careless approach to their treatments. If we didn't do anything else right in the office, I was determined that we would at least look the part.

In the mid-1980s I caved to persistent nurse requests and allowed white slacks and print tops. But I never wavered regarding the cap requirement. The stipulation was maintained – to the delight of my older patients – until the end of my private practice days.

Delivery Days

During my sixth month of practice, I decided to get back into obstetrics. My experience in the military had been a positive one, and deliveries would help build the practice. If a primary care physician delivered the baby, he usually assumed its care. There was only one board-certified pediatrician, Dr. McDermott, in town at the time.

I approached Dr. Joseph O'Neill, chief of the OB/GYN department and indicated my intentions. There was a hint of wariness in his response, but he voiced no objections. It was agreed that, with approval from the mother-to-be and Dr. O'Neill in attendance, I would deliver a couple of his patients.

The occasion of the first delivery I remember well. Dr. Manganaro, one of the senior general practitioners, provided the anesthesia: ether dripped onto a mesh cone covering the mother's mouth and nose. The amount given was determined by the color of the patient's nail beds. If pink, the anesthesia was continued; if blue, it was stopped.

Two trained anesthesiologists who could offer other anesthetic options were on staff, but physicians who had performed this appropriate but less-current procedure for years were not about to be dislodged. The delivery went well. During the procedure Dr. O'Neill muttered a few words which had the cadence of a curse. *Perhaps*, I thought, *he's just religious*. A fine-looking baby boy was delivered. The mother's smile conveyed her pleasure.

Turning toward Dr. O'Neill, I noticed a bead of sweat on his brow and – possibly because of the angle of the overhead light – a look of relief in his eyes. A circumcision, with a Gomco clamp, completed the evening's work.

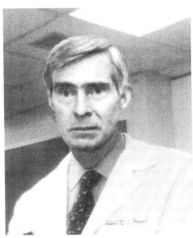

Joseph O'Neill, M.D. Obstetrician/
Gynecologist

After another delivery, with the good Dr. O'Neill standing by, I was granted privileges in obstetrics.

For approximately three years I had an active obstetric practice. Tuesday was our OB day in the office. However, as the general medicine area of the practice became busier, daytime deliveries caused significant disruptions in the schedule; those occurring at night made the following day a long one. For these reasons, a very satisfying part of my practice was gradually phased out.

Good Intentions Gone Awry

Elsie, our secretary, had proved to be a positive addition to the practice. A longtime resident of South County, she knew many of the patients and provided a comfortable introduction to the office. This familiarity could have created a confidentiality problem – a situation we discussed – and to my knowledge there were never any breeches of patient information. Early to work and meticulous in appearance, she was a friendly phone presence whom I felt lucky to have on my staff.

My confidence in her led to laxity on my part. My habit at the end of each day was to match the receipts for the day against the charges on the day sheet. No discrepancies were ever noted, and as a result, my checks became less frequent. But when I did pay attention, I noticed that patients I knew I had seen that day were not listed on the sheet. It became apparent that Elsie hadn't entered their names, which allowed her to pocket their cash payments. It happened infrequently and the amounts certainly weren't large.

When confronted, she admitted her guilt, saying that the money was used to help support her grandkids. She was discharged. I didn't involve the police. In her early seventies, Elsie promised not to seek further employment – an unfortunate conclusion for a woman whom I had been pleased to have on my staff.

The Past Meets the Present

One autumn day, I received a call from John Paul Jones, M.D. requesting a meeting. Though a legend in the history of South County Hospital, we had never met, but I had heard he was retiring. Recalling our chat, I hope I didn't come across as the brash new kid on the block, prone to flip comments, rather than someone respectful of a physician who, by 1970, had spent sixty years serving the medical needs of the community. The inscription on his memorial stone, tucked into a small garden in front of the hospital, identifies him as the Founder of the South County Hospital Medical Staff.

We got together at his home on Kenyon Avenue. The square, two-story structure with its brick exterior was at odds with its shingled neighbors. Two small gardens, absent flowers, flanked the front door. The front lawn was free of colorful vegetation.

A small man in a dark suit and tie, with neatly-parted gray hair and eyes bright behind wire-rimmed glasses, greeted me with a handshake. I followed him into a sparsely furnished living room where we sat across from each other at a table with grooves available for storing gambling chips. Hands clasped before him, carriage erect, he thanked me for coming by.

After a few questions about my practice thus far and how my family was acclimating to their new home, he got to the reason for the meeting.

"I saw your advertisement in the *Narragansett Times*," he began. "You're the first new blood we've had around here for a while." He smiled. "I guess you know I've been doing this job for a few years."

I nodded.

"Well, I've decided it's about time I officially called it a day. The few patients I have left need a bright young fellow like you, not an old grouch who is beginning to get very forgetful. So I'd like to hand over what I have left of my practice to you."

"Thank you," I said. "I'd be delighted to see them, but the problem will be, Dr. Jones, they may refuse to see me. Probably rather just hang on, hoping you change your mind."

He waved my comment away. "I'm putting an ad in the *Times* next week notifying everyone about the transfer of their records. That should put to rest any hanging-on talk. Yes, some of these families I've taken care of for over fifty years. It will be a shock to their systems, but they'll get over it."

Three large shoebox-shaped boxes were stacked on an adjoining couch. He asked me to bring one over. Inside were two stacks of index cards alphabetically listed with protruding tabs.

He randomly selected one of the cards and handed it to me. "Can you read my writing?"

Very precisely, in a cursive, scratchy style, were his office notes, seldom more than a half dozen lines for any visit. Most patients had multiple cards, stapled or secured by an elastic band.

"Yes, Sir, no problem."

A larger box on the floor was filled with instruments: scissors, scalpels, forceps, clamps, hemostat, and some I didn't recognize.

"Take these if you like," he said. "You'll probably never bother with them. All used back in the dark ages."

As I poked through the collection, I asked him to identify one: a flat board from which projected six metal blades. On the other side of the board, a small lever was attached to a spring.

Dr. Jones smiled. "That goes back to the bloodletting days," he said. "It was still being done when I started out, along with leeches, and I still use it once in a while."

He demonstrated how it was used. The lever, when retracted, drew the blades into a cocked position. The flat side of the board was placed against the patient's skin. When the spring released, the blades shot out to about 1/8 inch, puncturing the skin and producing six bleeding points. These were wiped away and the procedure repeated at various sites on the body. He said a lot of people felt better a few days after the procedure. His theory: the multiple areas of inflammation caused a white blood cell response which neutralized whatever bacteria was causing the illness. A significant portion of Dr. Jones's medical career, it must be remembered, occurred during the pre-antibiotic era.

After the business portion of the visit was complete, we chatted. I asked him about the early days before there was a hospital.

"That's sort of an interesting story, Doctor," he replied. "Do you have a few minutes?"

I nodded that I had.

In a quiet, reedy voice, lubricated with frequent sips of water, he told his story.

"When I came to town, just after World War I, South County didn't have a hospital, nor were there any between Providence and New London. Patients who needed hospitalization were taken by horse-cart to the Kingston Train Station. When the next train to Providence came through – I think they ran three a day," he said, "the patient was put in a baggage car and transported to the city. From there an ambulance went to Rhode Island Hospital.

"In 1918, two events happened which really showed the need for a local hospital. A young Narragansett boy died of a perforated appendix. Actually happened on the train taking him to the city. A few days later, Caroline Hazard, an extremely well-to-do lady, came to see me. Her family owned the textile mills in Peace Dale. She told me her brother had been ill recently. They had called his doctor in Providence, and it took him a full day to get down here. 'My brother almost died,' she said. 'He was operated on right in the house.'

"'Dr. Jones,' she said to me, 'we must have a hospital in South County. I want you to get together with the other physicians and decide what will be required.' There was only one other in the area–Dr. Henry Potter – so that was easy. We thought it was a great idea. I got back to Caroline and discussed what was needed. With her wealth and connections – and determination – a seven-bed cottage hospital opened in 1919. Right here, on Kenyon Avenue, down the street. The house is still there."

"What a story, Dr. Jones. I never knew."

"We've come a long way. To give you an idea of the population at the time – my telephone number was three. Police and fire were one and two. He shook his head. I can't believe the changes that have happened around here and in medicine since back then. I would love to be starting off again like you are." The doctor slowly got to his feet. "Anyway, the best of luck, young man. I have some wonderful patients. Take good care of them for me."

"Yes, I will, Doctor. Thank you," I said.

I thought it a poignant moment. Sixty years of practice – the surgeries, the deliveries, the thousands of patients that had filled his medical lifetime, reduced to three boxes of cards and a bunch of discolored instruments.

Dr. Jones saw me to the door. We shook hands.

"Would it be all right if I dropped by when I need advice on any of your patients?" I asked.

His face brightened. "By all means, Dr. McKee, please do. I would like that."

I carried the remnants of the doctor's career to my car. The evening was cool, a wan sun casting its last shadows, the day coming to a close. The setting, it seemed, fit the moment.

Dr. Jones died in 1980, six days before his ninety-third birthday.

South County Hospital - Beginnings and Beyond

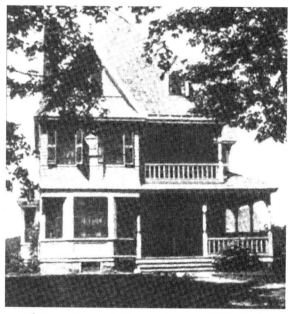

Cottage Hospital, Kenyon Avenue, Wakefield

The cottage hospital served the community for six years. It was also the residence for Dr. Jones, his wife and daughter. They occupied the major portion of the first floor, while the remainder was configured into a reception/waiting area and three examination rooms. The operating room on the second floor was also used for obstetrics. A small nursery adjoined. The third floor had two bedrooms for nurses who might be doing private duty. Mrs. Jones served as nurse and receptionist and administered anesthesia. Thirteen hundred patients were treated there during its operation.

Before the cottage hospital celebrated its third anniversary, it became apparent that the facility was overextended, lacking the space and faculties to adequately serve a growing population. A committee was formed, which after deliberation formally petitioned the town for a grant of land to establish an entity to be known as South County Hospital.

A tract of land at the end of Kenyon Avenue, known as "the poor farm" (a building and garden that offered food and shelter to those in need), was identified. The request was granted, construction begun by the Lois Bell Company, and in November 1925, the 42-bed South County Hospital, at a cost of $250,000, was dedicated. Caroline Hazard – having contributed $50,000 to the project – was named chairman of the hospital board and Dr. Jones, superintendent.

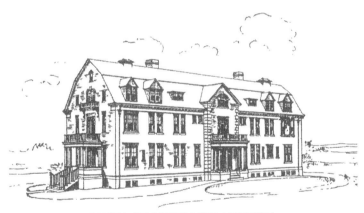

SOUTH COUNTY'S NEW HOSPITAL

Angell & Swift, Providence, Architects   Stevens & Lee, Boston, Consultants

With the "poor farm" closed, the indigent population utilized the Oliver Watson Home in West Kingston, which offered similar services.

As with any new venture, a considerable period passed before income from hospital services covered expenses. The concerted efforts of the South County community during that period were instrumental in addressing the shortfall. All manner of hospital fundraising events were held locally. Wakefield business owners donated time, money, and services; substantial philanthropy was continued by the more affluent of the population.

An example of cooperative involvement: a room in the hospital was designated the Preserve Room, which housed a series of shelves. Each had a label affixed, identifying the townships served – Wakefield, Narragansett, North Kingstown, Matunuck, and Kingston. Each town was responsible for keeping their shelf stocked with foodstuffs. Often this took the form of preserved foods, hence the name, but perishables were also welcomed. Patients' meals were provided in this manner for a number of years, as were linens for the hospital beds.

Nurse staffing became a problem; few were available locally. Most nurses were trained and lived in Providence. Travel time between the city and South County was measured in hours, and few were willing to spend that much time in transit. With funding provided by the Bacon family, a building was erected next to the hospital which offered lodging for nurses. This inducement and the reasonable rent – $7.50 a week with meals – brought enough nurses to the area to alleviate the staffing deficit. During the 1960s, another nursing shortage necessitated the use of medics stationed at the Quonset Point Naval Air Station. At one point, sixteen naval corpsmen were living in the Bacon house while working at the hospital.

In 1952 the Hazard Memorial Wing was completed, increasing beds by 14 and enlarging service areas. In 1962 new laboratories, a surgical suite, and 11 more beds were added.

At the time of my arrival in 1970, the first floor of the hospital served a mixed medical, surgical population with private and semi-private rooms. Pediatrics, obstetrics, and the nursery occupied the second floor. The third floor, primarily used for medical patients, featured an open porch with a southern exposure and Salt Pond view. Patients were frequently brought out on fine days to enjoy the sun and fresh air. This practice was discontinued a few years later when the structural integrity of the porch came into question. Radiology, surgical services, and the room used for emergencies, were located on the basement floor.

The Borda Wing, designed for the post-acute patient, had opened one month earlier. This, the third expansion of the hospital, featured larger, more patient-friendly rooms (at less the usual room charge) and brought the in-patient capacity to 100 beds.

An intensive care unit was not in place at the time. Dr. John Brady, a Mayo Clinic-trained internist, joined the staff in 1970. Under his direction, a three-bed unit was opened on the first floor adjacent to the nurses' station, and in the process, lidocaine was introduced (the first anti-arrhythmic in the hospital formulary).

The evolution of South County Hospital continued in a steady, incremental fashion. As the 1970s unfolded, the essential components – laboratory, radiological and clinical services – were equivalent to any community hospital in the state.

A Benign Dictator

The president and CEO of the hospital in 1970 was Donald Ford. Mr. Ford – whom I never addressed otherwise until he was no longer associated with the hospital– had been in that position since 1958. His was an interesting background.

Fourteen years of his life were spent with the Alexian Brothers, a contemplative religious order formed in Belgium during the fourteenth century. Over time, their mission had evolved to providing care for the sick and destitute. During his years with the brothers, Don became a registered nurse, worked as a hospital administrator, and earned a degree in nursing education. Subsequent to leaving the order – following a rather circuitous route – he became chief executive officer of South County Hospital.

During his reign, Mr. Ford shepherded the facility from backwater obscurity to one that merited comparison with any

Rhode Island hospital, through improvement of the physical plant, expansion of services, and increased membership of medical staff.

Don's style meshed perfectly with the down-home, courtly-mannered, middle-class population of South County. The intelligence and palaver of his Irish heritage fit well the integrity and common sense of the Yankee population, a cohort which comprised a significant part of the southern Rhode Island demographic.

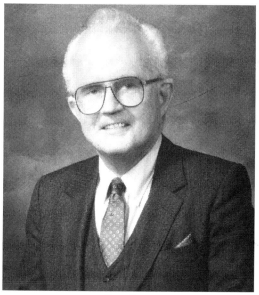

Don Ford
CEO of South County Hospital (1958 - 1986)

When chatting with Mr. Ford on hospital business, I always sensed a wariness, an appraising look in his eyes that accompanied his ready smile. He was on the lookout, it seemed, for a hidden agenda, as though he had been outsmarted once or twice and was not about to let it happen again.

An encounter we had in the early days of my practice illustrates Mr. Ford's typical approach to a situation and his method of resolution.

Physicians were (and presumably still are) notoriously tardy in dictating summaries on their discharged patients. This presented a problem for the medical records department for a variety of reasons (insurance company requests would be one example). A tedious and frustrating exercise ensued, involving multiple phone calls to the doctor's office and notes left in their mailboxes. Once the efforts of the department had reached the no-recourse-left level, Mr. Ford was notified.

One busy afternoon, my secretary knocked on the door of an examining room and informed me that Mr. Ford was on the phone and wanted to speak with me.

"Tell him I'll call him when I get a chance," I said.

A moment later the knock was repeated. "Mr. Ford said he'd appreciate it if you could take his call now," my secretary said, with a shrug of her shoulders.

I excused myself to the patient and went to the phone. "Yes, Mr. Ford?"

"I know you're busy," he answered. "Only take a minute." And with that he began to chat, even offered a joke. He asked me about my aunt, whom he knew. I was fidgeting at the end of the line. I mentioned I was in the middle of seeing patients.

"Oh, of course. My apologies." He paused. His voice took on a dry and measured tone. "I'm told, Dr. McKee, that your discharge summaries are overdue."

"Yes, Mr. Ford, I'll get them done. Next day or so."

"Are you wearing a watch, Dr. McKee?"

"Yes, Mr. Ford."

"What time does it say?"

"One-forty."

Mr. Ford cleared his throat. "You will have your overdue records completed by five o'clock today." There was no jocularity or hint of compromise in his voice.

"I'll still be working in the office, Mr. Ford."

"Then by all means, do as you wish. But realize, if they aren't completed by that time, you will no longer have admitting privileges at South County Hospital." He paused. "Do you understand?"

"Yes, Mr. Ford."

"Good. Nice chatting with you. Say hello to your aunt for me." The line went dead.

The dictations were completed by 4:45. That was the last conversation I had with Mr. Ford in that regard.

Success in business, it is said, is determined by the quality of the people who advise the CEO. The talented people Mr. Ford made part of his administration are a testament to that wisdom: Edna Otto, RN, with a master's degree in nursing, was the chief nurse; Bob Menard, a financial whiz whom Ford whisked away from Blue Cross/Blue Shield to become CFO; and Ralph Misto, who rose from director of laboratories to chief of patient services (and some years later, president of the hospital).

Though not unduly modest, if Mr. Ford were to recap his accomplishments at the hospital, he would probably gloss over his contributions to discuss the efforts of the staff and his hard-working management team. To dismiss further conversation, he'd likely trot out a joke: "This Irishman walked into a hospital one day..."

Yankees - Swamp and Otherwise

Patients reflect the cultural idiosyncrasies of their locale and Rhode Island has its own unique population. The term Yankee has been used to describe a notable component of South County. Their position as the predominant ethnic entity in the community has become diminished over the decades by the influx of other nationalities and inter-marriage between groups. Before all vestiges of their influence and prominence have faded, a mention should be made of their background.

The origin of the term "Yankee" is in dispute. The most reasonable suggestion of the many offered: it was the closest phonetic equivalent to the Native American word for English.

In the north-eastern states, Yankee refers specifically to those of colonial ancestry, descendants of the original settlers. During the early days, they typically lived in villages consisting of clusters of small farms; in South County many fished commercially. Education was emphasized and many went on to become teachers, bankers, merchants, and as the years passed, some became prominent in the higher reaches of government and commerce. Many of the mills in New England –including the complex in Peace Dale– were owned and operated by Yankees.

A stereotype of the Yankee developed: frugal, honest, hardworking, with a common sense approach to life and its problems. "Yankee ingenuity" and "get up and go" were aphorisms commonly applied. God-fearing Congregationalists, they were the moral and cultural arbiters of many New England towns.

Another group from the same gene pool but culturally a world apart was the "Swamp Yankee." They also had fled England but their exit, in most instances, had little to do with religious freedom or lofty aspirations. If not a member of the boat crew or indentured servants travelling with their owners, they were probably fleeing some misconduct charge or legal difficulty in England. Most lacked a formal education and had little desire to pursue one.

The derivation of the "swamp" portion of their nickname remains obscure. One theory: lacking the social graces, resources, and ambitions of those living in the more stable, cultured communities, they were evicted and forced to live in the less desirable swamp areas. Another notion: when under attack by Indians, rather than stay and fight, they ran and hid in the swamps.

They did share many of the qualities of their better situated brethren: fiercely loyal, independent, stubborn, laconic, didn't suffer fools easily, spoke their mind, and were able to wrest a living from the land and the sea.

But their vision didn't extend beyond the fields they worked or the waters they fished. Although they shared the same roots as the Brahmin bluebloods and were in America for an equivalent period of time, they never aspired to success, fame or fortune.

"Swamp Yankees" have been compared to rednecks in the southern states, who also have established their own identity, a lifestyle apart from the mainstream. They, too, like their music country, their beer Bud, their tractors Deere, and their women, (like their Ford 150s), well built. The only difference: their pick-up trucks fly the confederate flag.

The Physician You Know...

In 1970 there was a cadre of older physicians, members of the hospital staff for a considerable period, most in excess of twenty years. The first wave of doctors from the post-World War II era, they had come on the heels of the originals (Drs. Jones and Potter). Fine gentlemen all, they established something of a fiefdom in the institution. With a voting majority they controlled the medical agenda, determined physician privileges and designated department chiefs and committee chairs. As might be assumed, they were not keen on functions they had performed for years being assumed by newcomers. (For instance: Dr. Attilio Manganaro in his anesthesia role and Dr. Clifford Hathaway, a Harvard-trained physician, who performed all in-patient electrocardiograms.)

The hospital did not own an EKG machine when I joined the staff. Dr. Hathaway brought in his own office apparatus, encased in a rich, walnut-stained, rectangular box. After he ran the tracing, he'd contact the ordering physician with the results. Unfortunately, the machine frequently became inoperable. With these interruptions and an internist (Dr. John Brady) added to the staff, the hospital purchased their own machine and eventually took over the service.

Most of these physicians also provided obstetric and pediatric care for their patients and performed their own surgeries. When Dr. John Walsh joined the staff in 1946, he was the hospital's first board-certified surgeon. Trained at Boston City Hospital, Jack, as he was called, was available to assume – along with Dr. Mauricio Goldberg – the lead surgeon role, when requested by the general practice providers who were expected to assist at the surgery. That framework, in place for many years, had well served both the community and the physicians involved. Alterations were not considered necessary nor warmly welcomed.

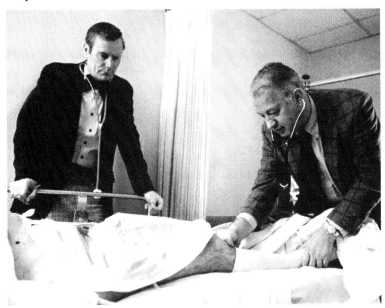

Dr. Mauricio Goldberg, surgeon, with author at South County Hospital

As physicians resisted change, so too, did patients. For generations the general practitioner — a trusted, familiar presence — had taken care of their families, from operations to treating sore throats, fixing broken bones, and delivering their kids. That kind of bond was not easily broken, especially in a population where trust wasn't bestowed easily.

That was the situation the "Young Guns," as they were called in some quarters, found themselves in when they came to town in the mid-1960s. They included Dr. Bob Conrad, surgeon; Dr. Joseph O'Neill obstetrician/gynecologist; and Dr. Bill McDermott, pediatrician – the first board-certified physicians to join the staff since Dr. Walsh. They were the new kids on the block and the vanguard of change which in the upcoming decade would transform the delivery of medicine, both nationally and in our little corner of the world.

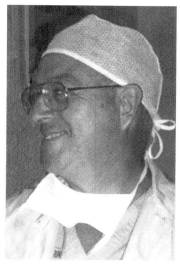

Dr. Robert Conrad, surgeon,
South County Hospital

Their acceptance by the community and the entrenched physician bloc in the hospital took time. Afternoons were spent reading medical journals, waiting for the phone to ring. But competence can't be denied. When I arrived in May of 1970, their practices were prospering.

The key to the turnaround were the nurses. Working with practitioners on a daily basis they could readily sift through the externals to recognize the physician both competent and current in his field. Their recommendation of a doctor to family and friends – the seal of approval – was a physician's best advertisement. That started the ball rolling. To quote Dr. Conrad, "The nurses saved my ass."

A Breakthrough

At the time of Don Ford's retirement from South County Hospital, having served twenty-eight years at the helm, he was asked to identify the ten most important changes during his tenure. One he chose was the appointment of Larry Bouchard, an osteopathic physician (DO), to the staff in 1963, the first such acceptance by an allopathic (MD-staffed), hospital in Rhode Island.

The differences between the two disciplines involved philosophy, training, and treatment. Osteopathy took a more holistic approach, looking at the whole person in the process of diagnosis, whereas the MD focused more on specific signs and symptoms. The training of the osteopath included an emphasis on muscular-skeletal manipulative procedures, not a focus of the allopathic curriculum: the MD treated primarily with prescription medications, whereas the osteopath preferred manipulation techniques and preventative medical measures.

Dr. Rod Urquhart had an osteopathic practice in Wakefield during the 1940s and 50s but was never associated with SCH. Cranston General, established in 1933, was the base of operations for the osteopathic physician community in Rhode Island.

The differences today are mainly historical. Allopathic and osteopathic physicians work together in hospitals across the country without discernible differences in diagnostic and treatment approaches.

During his early years of practice, Dr. Bouchard had no professional connection with South County Hospital, nor were his requisitions for lab or X-ray services for his patients honored there. In spite of these impediments, Dr. Bouchard's practice prospered. Mr. Ford, learning of this and perhaps recognizing a neglected revenue source, contacted Larry and informed him that the restrictions had been lifted.

A year or so later, Mr. Ford called again, suggesting that Larry apply for staff privileges. The hospital board of trustees was aware of and in agreement with the offer. Dr. Bouchard's application, when brought before the medical staff for a vote, was soundly rejected. The only votes in Larry's favor came from the "young guns" and one of the senior physicians. However, the trustees, in a rare use of their authority in physician matters, overruled the doctors' decision and in July, 1968 granted Dr. Bouchard staff privileges. It should be noted that when staff re-appointments came around again, Larry's application was accepted unanimously by the staff.

An active member of the American Osteopathic Association, Dr. Bouchard assumed various positions of responsibility, culminating in the presidency of their national organization in 1993. Larry was also one of fifty physicians appointed to an advisory board created by President Clinton in his attempt to implement a national health care program.

Dr. Bouchard paved the way for a number of osteopathic physicians, representing all major specialties, who have joined the hospital staff over the years. (The first cardiologist at South County, Dr. Robert McGhee, was an osteopathic physician.)

Larry and I shared coverage for many years, and the loyalty and trust he inspired in his patients was extraordinary. In some quarters it was felt that Larry, although an outstanding physician, had missed his true calling — as a stand-up comedian. A shaggy-dog example: a man fell into a rug-making machine, his widow then bought the rug which contained her husband and put it in the living room. One night her new boyfriend was walking across the carpet...and the story goes on from there. After fifty-two years of dedicated service to the good folk of South County, Larry retired. A short time later, in 2015, he passed away.

Colorful Characters

In any group there are those individuals more easily remembered, their recollection often accompanied by a smile or a shake of the head.

The South County Hospital physician ensemble during the 1970s was no different. It is to be emphasized that the instances described here are not related to medical proficiency, but rather personality and idiosyncrasy.

There resided in Narragansett a physician who felt that many maladies were a result of improper footwear. The poorly structured sandal, the unlaced loafer, and most significantly, any shoe that bound feet too tightly were the usual suspects. His advice to many of his patients was to buy properly constructed shoes, at least a size larger than those presently worn — and which were available for purchase from the doctor. It was related to me that often, at the time of the visit, the doctor cut out portions of the shoes the patient was wearing to illustrate the areas of concern, making his advice less a suggestion than a necessity.

This physician said he had gained this insight as a child. His frequent headaches were abolished when his mother bought him — as a practical measure — shoes larger than usual so he could "grow into them." He applied this concept to other medical conditions with success. He had a loyal following, quite willing to walk the miles in his shoes.

I knew of one Wakefield physician with a robust practice who seldom wrote prescriptions. Medications were dispensed color-coded to match the acuity of the presenting illness, with yellow indicating the least serious and red the most. Other hues identified gradations between. The ingredients of the medications were never revealed to the patients. They grasped, however, the trajectory of their illness by the color of the pills given them. Red to green, for instance, identified improvement.

The placebo effect is present to varying degrees when any medication is taken. Just being told a prescription will help triggers a positive response. Various studies have demonstrated this. It has also been shown that when colored (especially red) sugar tablets or capsules are substituted for the white variety, the placebo effect is appreciably enhanced. Present-day pharmaceutical companies, hoping to market a new pain medication, must submit double-blind studies to the FDA and gain approval before their medication can be used by the general public. Frequently the companies have found – to their chagrin – that subjects receiving the placebo are obtaining pain relief to the extent that there isn't a statistically significant difference between the placebo and the drug being marketed. So perhaps our Wakefield physician was on to something.

Another interesting physician on staff was Dr. Al Gobeille, Jamestown's only doctor for many years. My first sighting of the gentleman occurred on a summer afternoon in the ER.

Striding through the door was a tall, lean man, his skin a Coppertone brown. His shaven bald scalp, also tan, glistened in the overhead lights. A sun-faded, light blue shirt, unbuttoned to mid-chest, exposed a gold chain and a hairless chest. Casual white boating pants, encircled at the waist by a length of cord, reached to sock-free feet and sandals. Completing the ensemble was an unlit cheroot jauntily jutting from the corner of his mouth and a stethoscope slung around his neck. Not known to me at the time: his preferred mode of transport was a Harley D with short pipes.

Al, a Tufts medical school alum, marched to his own drummer, as everything about him would suggest. With a practice somewhat removed from the South County area, he was an intermittent presence this side of the bridge. I frequently covered his ER rotation and as a result got to know him fairly well. If I could place Al — with his restlessness, his resistance to conformity, a free spirit chained to a structured profession — with a group that best fit his persona, it would be the surfing community. If born twenty-five years later, Al would have been the ultimate surfer dude.

The medical needs of the people of Jamestown were ably served by Dr. Gobeille for well over two decades. His eventual departure from the island was greeted with dismay and disbelief. I acquired a few of his patients who told me up front that I was their interim provider until the good Dr. G returned.

As he would freely admit, Al liked the ladies — and to complete the synergy – the ladies liked him. Tales could be told. He eventually married the considerably younger, third-floor ward secretary at SCH. Al found some acreage deep in the woods of Maine on which he built their log cabin home and where, according to her father, they lived happily and well.

The Nightingales

Over the years I've encountered nurses whom I'd worked with in the past. I'm struck – especially by those of more mature vintage – by their nostalgia for "the good old days," which for them (and for me) meant the years between the early 1960s and the mid-1980s. Their reminiscences are speckled with anecdotes: Nurse Ratched supervisors, cranky patients, their own "Dr. Kildares" (Dr. McDreamy for the younger reader), clinical mishaps, outdated procedures, lecherous physicians – the OR assignations, the library trysts – the good, the bad, and the bizarre. These flashbacks, remembered with mellowed hindsight, bring a laugh and on occasion, a tear. Nurses, as much as any group, can appreciate and feel amazed at the changes that have taken place in their profession.

Recollecting her days as director of Surgical Services at South County Hospital through that era, Barbara Hackey, RN, remembered the technological and specialist deficits. "There was one X-ray room, no MRIs, no CAT scans or ultrasound," she told the *Narragansett Times* in 1974. "The surgeon who took your gall bladder out one day might set your arm the next. Everybody did everything." She, too, decried the loss of the professional "aura" represented by the traditional white uniform. "These days it's impossible to tell a doctor from a nurse, a nurse from a technician."

Doctors' attire in those early days also befit their professional status. Most physicians – certainly the older group – wore suits or jackets with ties. There was no mistaking the physician in a hospital line-up.

The most significant nurse/physician interaction occurred during patient rounds. They were traditionally accomplished in the morning. Surgeons, due to early operating room schedules, would often defer to a later time. A certain formality was involved. Arriving on the floor, the doctor was greeted by the head nurse with a, "Good morning, Sir." The charts for his patients had been placed in a mobile rack. After the usual pleasantries and perhaps a chat about a patient of particular concern, rounds began. At the bedside, the nurse summarized the pertinent observations noted during the past twenty-four hours. It was a good time for any doctor to pay close attention.

The wisdom of doing so was made clear to me when toiling as an intern at Pawtucket Memorial Hospital. The chief of medicine at the time, Dr. Ed Lovering, conducted Grand Rounds each Friday morning. In his entourage were the senior and junior residents, interns, students, and the head nurse on the floor.

Discussion of a patient always included a nursing assessment. In fact, Dr. Lovering insisted each case begin with that input.

One day a student, in an off-hand comment overheard by Dr. Lovering, said that more attention was paid to the comments from the nurse during rounds than the doctors.

Dr. Lovering turned to him. "Young man, let me tell you something. Any doctor who doesn't pay attention to what nurses say, who feels he doesn't need their help, is doing so at his own peril. And if you don't talk to them, at least read their notes. I may spend thirty minutes with a patient. They're with them twenty-four hours a day." The advice continued; the good doctor was on a roll. The focus of Dr. Lovering's rant stood silently, shoulders slumped, hands pushed deep into the pockets of his white coat as he lamented his unfortunate aside.

I also learned that if you demeaned a nurse or for whatever reason got on her bad side, your hospital life would henceforth be miserable. Another profession should be considered. The "hell hath no fury" dictum kicked in – and not just from the affronted nurse, but also the network of colleagues from other floors who collaborated with equivalent zeal.

Rounds completed, the doctor wrote orders for his patients. A sampling of available medications from the late '60s and early '70s would include:

> Gastric: antacids, tincture of belladonna, cimetidine
>
> Hypertension: reserpine, hydrochlorothiazide, beta blockers
>
> Cardiac: nitroglycerine and amyl nitrate for angina, quinidine as an anti-arrhythmic, digoxin for congestive heart failure
>
> Psychotropics: chlorpromazine, meprobamate
>
> Antibiotics: penicillin, streptomycin, sulfonamides

Other orders might be included, some of which are seldom seen today:

- Sippy diet – hourly milk and cream feedings with large doses of antacids
- Dangle legs 15 minutes, three times a day – a stage in the progression of increased activity, usually after a cardiac event
- Buck's traction – pull is exerted on the lower extremities by a system of ropes, weights and pulleys, used in hip and femoral fractures
- Semi-Fowler bed position – the head of the bed placed at an angle of usually forty-five degrees to relax abdominal muscles and improve breathing
- Three H enema (high, hot, and a helluva lot)

- Ambulate patient 15 minutes, three times a day
- May have cigarette after meals on porch
- Glass of wine or single beer with meals (family will supply)
- Rotate tourniquets as necessary – procedure in which tourniquets were applied to the extremities in order to reduce the volume of blood returning to a compromised heart muscle

Having been confronted in the past with the hieroglyphics of a physician's scrawl, the wise nurse reviewed with the doctor all medication orders. Better now than when a sound-alike medication or a misplaced period had triggered an untoward event.

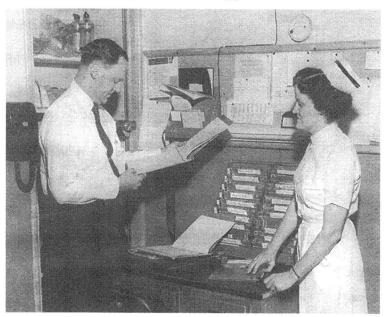

Dr. John Walsh in 1972

Rounds completed, the physician thanked the nurse for her help, indicated where he could be reached, and if not on call, the name of the covering physician.

This recitation of the rounds ritual is offered as a tintype of how things were done 45 years ago, not an intimation that the old way was the better way. The goal – improvement of the physical status of the patient – has not changed, but a ubiquitous technology has transformed the process, from history-taking and nursing plans, to the way medications are dispensed. The concern for nurses working in this electronic environment: becoming estranged from the patient, jeopardizing the human connection. (The patient complaint: "The nurse spends more time looking at the computer screen than at me," is not an isolated observation.) That alliance – often the key determinant when patients rank hospital quality of care – is as essential and efficacious now as it was for Nurse Florence back in her day.

A Legend in His Time

One morning during the first week of my practice, the secretary from the office across the hall brought a gift – a pen and pencil set and a desk blotter – from her boss, Charles Farrell, M.D. "The doctor is away," she said, "but asked me to pass on his best wishes as you start your practice in South County. He is looking forward to meeting you."

Dr. Farrell was one of the senior attending physicians at Memorial Hospital when I was in training there. During the latter years of his practice he operated a clinic in Pawtucket, R.I. at a time when that concept was not commonplace; in fact, his was one of the first in the state. Now in his seventies, he had sold the clinic, moved to Narragansett, and opened an office. (His daughter Betty Ann, her husband Tom, and their brood of eight, lived in the former Cottage Hospital in Wakefield.)

When we did meet a short time later (his remembrance of me was vague), his appearance had scarcely altered over the approximately five years. Gray hair cut short (parted neatly), and skin stretched taut over a fold-free face were as remembered. A fastidious dresser, I had never seen him attired in anything other than a suit and tie.

"Came down here to take it easy for a while," he told me. "See a few patients a week. Ease into retirement. But now," he said, "I'm busier than ever. Glad to have you across the hall. Hope you don't mind if I pass some patients on to you."

I assured him I would be delighted.

Politically astute, over the course of his career, Charlie had been President of the R.I Medical Society, the state representative to the American Medical Society (AMA), and the president of the R.I. chapter of the American Academy of Family Practice. Although a stalwart opponent of government's intrusion into the private practice of medicine (Medicare), he had accepted the inevitable. At our staff meetings he gamely attempted to translate the minutiae of the law into terms more palatable to his generally intractable colleagues. Not an easy sell.

Over the next few years, Dr. Farrell and I became friendly. During our chats he would speak of his career (he initially trained to be a dentist), the missteps made, and the successes enjoyed over the years. What I thought interesting: in both scenarios the stories were often presented as cautionary tales; success, he inferred, could be as damaging as failure.

Of course, there were the war stories. You couldn't be in practice as long as Charlie (approaching 60 years) and not have a quiver full of vignettes at your disposal. One I remember as a particular favorite.

Some background: An aggressive modality used in the treatment of acute, life-threatening heart failure was phlebotomy or venesection. In this procedure, 300-500 cc's of blood were removed from the vascular system. The antecubital veins in the arm were commonly used. The improvement in a patient's condition with the decrease in volume was often spectacular.

Historical aside: *George Washington died in 1799 following removal of 1.7 liters of blood during a bloodletting procedure. It was later determined that the president had an epiglottitis (a condition in which the flap which covers the windpipe swells and blocks the flow of air to the lungs.)*

Dr. Farrell related the following story: At Mass one Sunday morning, a distraught lady, a patient of his, burst into the church, found the doctor, and told him to come with her immediately. Her husband couldn't breathe and was dying.

He followed the lady to a nearby house. In the bedroom, her husband, a large man, was pushed upright in bed, pillows at his back, gasping for air, his face blue and swollen, neck veins distended, a look of terror on his face. Dr. Farrell did not have his medical bag with him but realized the man was in heart failure and drowning in fluid that had accumulated in his lungs.

"Get me the sharpest knife you have in the house and a few towels," he told the lady. "Someone call the ambulance. Also a couple pairs of women's stockings."

Pulling up the sleeves of the man's pajamas, he took a large carving knife and slashed the swollen antecubital veins at the bend of each elbow. Blood spurted onto the bed and "all over my suit," and continued to flow for a couple of minutes. Dr. Farrell fashioned tourniquets with the stockings and placed them around the man's arms and legs to reduce the flow of blood to the failing heart. The blood was mopped up with the towels.

By the time the ambulance arrived, the man – less distressed – was transported to the hospital. Dr. Farrell followed. The patient survived. The suit wasn't as fortunate.

Dr. Farrell continued in practice well into his 80s. Failing health eventually brought an end to his extraordinary career. The pen and paper set he gave me back in 1970 has long been lost but the desk blotter remains: right beneath the legal pad on which I'm writing this recollection.

Big Brother Intrudes

South County's transition from country hospital to equivalency with their big-city colleagues, initiated in the late 1960s, blossomed with the advent of the new decade. A country bumpkin shedding his overalls had put on some store-bought, big-boy clothes.

The face of change began with the flow of medical expertise into the community: Drs. Fitzgerald, Chamorro, and Golberg, orthopedics; Drs. Hambly and Lee, general surgery; Drs. Chronley and Falconer, pediatrics; Drs. Brady and Kenneth Hathaway (Clifford was his granduncle), internal medicine; Drs. McBurney and Zeurner, urology; Drs.Wepman, Coghlin and Asher, ophthalmology; Dr. Suvari, hematology/oncology; Drs. Liang and Yogaratnam, anesthesia.

A major expansion of surgical services occurred with the addition of Drs. Judkins and Murdocco – board-certified ear, nose and throat (ENT) surgeons. A variety of ENT surgeries, head and neck procedures, endoscopies, and traumatic maxillofacial repairs – formerly transferred to other facilities – were now done in-house.

By the end of the decade, every major specialty except neurological services had full-time representation on the staff.

The provision of healthcare – how it's provided, who provides it, and how it's paid for – was forever altered with the incursion of the federal government into the healthcare business.

Medicare, a national social insurance program, was signed into law in 1965 by President Lyndon Johnson. The purpose of the legislation was to provide health insurance for Americans aged sixty-five or older, regardless of income or medical history. The majority of people in that age bracket, being charged up to three times more than younger people, had found it virtually impossible to obtain or afford insurance from private companies. Physician fees were calculated using criteria that established a reasonable charge.

From the hierarchical reaches of the American Medical Association (AMA) to the physician in the trenches, the consensus was: government should stay out of their business. By implementing the program, the doors to socialized medicine would be flung open with communism right around the corner. The more candid physicians might admit that the pre-determined physician fee structure was the major concern. Communism they could live with.

The advent of HMOs (health maintenance organizations) and particularly DRGs (diagnosis-related groups) added fuel to the fevered conversation.

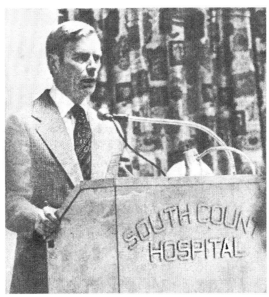

The author, as medical staff president, addressing the Board of Trustees and corporation members, annual meeting, 1978

DRGs are a federal payment system which reimburses hospitals for services, based on a classification of illnesses. The government had calculated the dollar value for each diagnosis, taking into account the patient's age and the services received during the hospital stay. If the costs to the facility were less than the amount allotted, they could keep the difference. However, if costs exceeded the DRG allowance, the hospital absorbed the discrepancy. The component of the plan that drew the most ire from physicians was the length-of-stay stipulation. If a patient hadn't been discharged within the prescribed time, hospital reviewers exerted significant pressure on the doctors to move them out. Arguments often ensued. Although the scenery, actors, and captions have changed, the same movie can be seen playing at any of your local hospitals to this day.

Dean of the Emergency Room

Among the new physicians who came on board in 1977 was Dr. Tim Drury. Prior to his affiliation with the hospital, he had served as medical director at the Wood River Health Services, a federally-funded facility in Hope Valley, R.I., deep in the heart of Yankee territory. Casual in dress and manner–– along with a backward-facing baseball cap, flip flops, and an ever-present Pittsburgh Steelers coffee mug – Tim was a tie-dyed bandana away from hippy status and not the type one would expect the "Yankees" to choose as their physician. But as with Al Gobeille in Jamestown, Tim's persona struck a chord. As one nurse who worked at the facility said, "They loved the guy." Personality and friendly banter aside, what attracted the folks of Hope Valley to Tim was more Yankee practical: the boy knew his medicine.

Tim came to SCH to work in the accident department (the emergency room): a windowless cubby on the basement floor; the exam room, a cleaned out storage space. Technology began and ended with an EKG machine. The radiology department, down the hall, was a reassuring resource. One nurse and a secretary completed the ER roster.

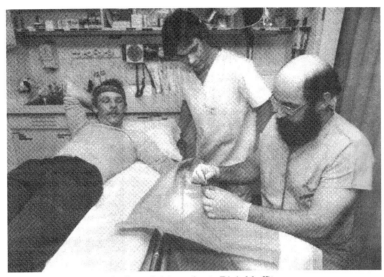

Left to right: patient; Rick Moffit,
physician assistant; and Dr. Tim Drury

Just as the setting was of another time, so too, were medications – the names of many scarcely recognized today. The same might be said of treatment procedures. Tim recalled the following instance from his early days at the hospital.

The gentleman presented in the accident room with a shoulder dislocation; he asked that his primary care physician be called. This was accomplished. His doctor arrived promptly and took the man into the examining room.

A few minutes later, Tim went in to offer assistance. On the floor, lying side-by-side, were the patient and doctor, their bodies facing opposite directions. The doctor was holding the arm with the dislocation, the heel of his shoeless foot deep into the armpit of the injured shoulder. Tim watched, the procedure new to him. As the doctor pulled the man's arm, he pushed with his heel, attempting to maneuver the errant head of the bone back to its normal position in the joint. Between efforts, he moved his foot from side-to-side, as though massaging the area.

"Anything I can do to help?" Tim asked.

"No, we're fine," the doctor answered. "Just have to work the spasm out of these muscles and it will pop back in. May take a few minutes."

The man walked out sometime later, shoulder in place, with instructions to wear a sling for a few days. The procedure was carried out without muscle relaxants or pain medication.

Reduction of a shoulder dislocation employing this technique dates back to ancient Greece and its use by Hippocrates (450 BC – 370 BC), so it has been around a while. The potential injury to the brachial plexus (a network of nerves located between the shoulder and neck which controls the muscles of the shoulder, arm, and hand), has discouraged its use. It also requires a certain dexterity which might be a challenge for some physicians.

Shortly thereafter, Dr. Drury, became board-certified in emergency medicine – one of the more physically demanding and mentally stressful medical specialties – and was appointed chief of the Emergency Department.

During our conversation, I made the observation (meant to provoke), that over the course of his career, technology had superseded the need for clinical acumen: EKG machines provided immediate interpretation, x-ray results a phone call away, comprehensive blood profiles available within the hour – or sooner if necessary – with an array of marvelous machines ready to provide the most precise information. The physician, I offered, was becoming little more than a translator of data to the patient.

Tim agreed that the computer had revolutionized the practice of medicine but protested and effectively rebutted my contention. He admitted, however, that the laying on of hands was a skill used less frequently to gather information. He provided an example. A physician, who worked in the Express

Care area in the ER, asked Tim to consult on a patient. The gentleman had presented with sharp chest wall pain and an irritating cough. Chest x-ray and cardiogram showed non-specific changes, a basic blood screen was normal. After a history review, Tim began his exam: ear, nose, and throat regions were acceptable; heart rate was quick but all cardiac sounds normal; breath sounds were shallow and a distinct pleural rub was heard in one lung field. The rest of the exam was non-revealing.

Approximately 65% of pleuritic rubs (inflammation of the lung linings which creates a grating sound when breaths are taken), are the result of a pulmonary emboli. Such was the case in this instance. The patient was admitted to the hospital. Why didn't the first physician pick up the abnormality? He didn't bother listening to the chest; in fact, he didn't carry a stethoscope, relying instead on the x-ray report. A lesson learned.

Tim retired in 2015 after nearly four decades in the trenches.

"You must be so glad, so ready," I said at the end of our chat, "to be finished with the twelve-hour days, the stress. All the Mickey Mouse crap you have to put up with in a position like that."

"I loved the job. Looked forward to my shifts."

I waited for the modifier, the punch line. There wasn't any. He meant it. *What a great thing to be able to say at the end of a long career. We all should be so lucky.*

Practices Grow

In my third year of practice, the business was building nicely. The modalities used by Dr. Squires in his office were replicated in mine, eventually including cardiac stress testing. The nurse took vital signs, prepared patients, ran EKGs, stuck fingers, dipped urine, and screened phone calls. A gem of a secretary performed multiple tasks – reception, phone, and insurance forms. Also, since I dictated notes on my patients, they had to be transcribed into each patient's chart by closing time. At this point I was seeing between twenty-five and thirty patients a day!

A misstep occurred when I opened a second office in Wickford, offering a late afternoon and evening schedule. The response was positive, and I took on a Navy physician stationed at the Quonset Point facility and expanded the hours. That arrangement worked well until the Navy base closed in 1974. My attempt to keep both offices going was not successful primarily because of an overlap of hours between the two offices. Dr. Bart Sanders, an excellent physician whom I worked with at the URI health services, took over the practice.

Another lesson learned during those early days: avoid wakes, especially when the guest of honor was your patient. I did attend on one occasion, the deceased being the father of a friend of mine. On entering the room where the body was being displayed, I was introduced to many in attendance as the doctor who took care of "Pa," lying stiff and stark in a casket a few feet away. Although well-intentioned, I don't think the identification– our respective images now forever linked– inspired a great deal of confidence in my doctoring skills. Certainly not the type of publicity one seeks when building a practice.

New Face in the Office

In April 1974 there was an addition to our office staff. Jack Cooke, whom I knew as an athletic trainer at URI, approached me and asked if I would consider bringing him into the practice. Jack was enrolled in Medex (Medicine Extension), a physician assistant program at Dartmouth College. He had completed the academic portion of the course, and in order to obtain his certification he was required to work under the supervision of a practicing physician for nine months.

We met and reviewed his medical background which, in the area of physical medicine and orthopedics, was extensive. Briefly, I described my practice and wondered what he could do for me that wasn't already being done by the nurse. He outlined aspects of care – routine physical examinations, as an example – that he thought would benefit the practice. Our talk ended with an introduction to my secretary and nurse. I asked him to call me the following afternoon.

My office colleagues offered no objections. When Jack called the next day, I welcomed him aboard.

In the 1970s the concept of the physician assistant, or PA, was in its infancy. In the state there were probably a half dozen, and none in South County. Dr. Charles Millard of Barrington was the first physician to employ one in Rhode Island, which at the time caused some consternation among the medical community.

The PA movement had its beginnings in 1965 when four Navy corpsmen were graduated from a program supervised by Dr. Eugene Stead at Duke University. His motivation in starting the program was to provide an adjunct to primary care providers whose ranks were diminishing, and to improve medical care for our rural populations. Dr. Stead incorporated many of the methods employed during World War II when medical students were "fast-tracked" through school to address the deficit of physicians in the military.

The Medex program was another pioneer in the PA movement. Their approach differed somewhat from the Duke model. Students entering the Medex program were required to have verifiable health care exposure – on the order of five years – prior to their application. The didactic portion of the program, although intense, was completed in three months. Students were expected to learn by doing, an "on the job" training approach which in Jack's instance was accomplished at my office.

The arrangement worked out well. A routine was established. Prior to my entering the exam room, and with the patient's permission, Jack took vital signs and a short history and made a physical assessment. As a medical student would, he presented the case to me, and after my evaluation we compared notes. The process proved as helpful for me as it was beneficial to him. While I was writing prescriptions, he was seeing the next patient.

Jack became familiar with and assisted in all office procedures. The nurse was delighted to have the help. Office disputes, turf issues, and personality conflicts were never a concern. The patients were delighted with the extra attention. Possessed of a great sense of Irish humor and an endless supply of bad jokes, Jack fit perfectly into our operation – a fortunate amalgam of four people who worked well together and enjoyed each other in the process.

Jack left us at the end of 1974, completed the program at Dartmouth, and became certified by the American Board of Physician Assistants the following year. A long, successful career – for which I take full credit – followed.

A Scent to Remember

My most acute recollections have always been sparked by smell. While the lilt of a laugh may invoke a memory for some, as a song lyric might for others, my trigger has always been a fragrance. The hint of perfume as a woman passes, the scent of lilac through an open window, the tang of salt from a stormy ocean, will invariably prompt a rush of memory. I now include Bengay in my list of olfactory souvenirs. It reminds me of Sue Alice.

The addition originated soon after my trusted confidante and office nurse par excellence married and left the practice and area. Her departure coincided with our move in 1980 to a new location on Holley Street in Wakefield.

Dr. Jaime Chamorro (an orthopedic surgeon), and I had partnered in the construction of a professional building at that site. A two-story structure, we each had an office on the upper level. Over the years, a variety of tenants occupied the lower space. The location was excellent and the building designed to our liking, each suite fashioned to our practice needs. An exciting project from conception to completion.

Three weeks into our new digs, the nurse vacancy remained unfilled. Productivity and peace of mind were jeopardized. When two of the more promising applicants decided not to take the position, a hint of desperation crept into my interviews.

The session with Sue Alice, however, went well. Pert, young, enthusiastic, and appropriately nervous, she offered a background as a phlebotomist and ECG tech, with a myriad of complimentary references. Twisting the end of the long ponytail that curled over her shoulder, she avowed a lifelong interest in office nursing. The chat was interrupted by a series of sneezes stifled with a handful of tissues; she had brought a large box of Kleenex with her. Sue Alice agreed to accept the position as soon as a replacement could be found for her present job. A sense of responsibility, I was pleased to note. Not a common thing these days.

Sue Alice handled her first day, a particularly hectic one, with aplomb and humor. I was struck by her ramrod posture and springy gait, which caused her long ponytail to bounce rhythmically off her back. Ballet, of course, I recollected from her resume.

The first scent of Bengay floated by toward the end of her second week. Sue Alice, though still efficient, seemed more withdrawn and less chatty than usual. I traced the aroma to her and asked what the problem was. With head frozen to her shoulders and eyes directed at me through quivering lashes, she explained that a particularly strenuous ballet session had caused a severe neck spasm. I offered a muscle relaxant, but she requested Fiorinal with Codeine. Though I preferred not to use narcotics for this condition, I acceded to her request and prescribed ten for the weekend. She responded well, and by Monday morning she was her usual mobile self again.

I didn't notice the Ace bandage until Wednesday, and only after she exchanged her nursing shoe for a pink slipper.

"Racquetball," she explained.

"Can you manage?"

"I'll try," she answered. Her lips were trembling.

All that sitting around with her legs elevated really worked. By Saturday afternoon her recovery was so complete, she felt she could enter a racquetball tournament the following day.

"Don't sprain the other one," my secretary joked as we left for the weekend.

Rather than the Bengay, it was the crutch that caught my attention the following week.

"Would you believe it?" she said, recounting details of the mishap to her other ankle.

Yes, she would do her "darnedest" to stay on the job, but, "Would it be all right if I rested once in a while between patients?" Though sympathetic, I felt a bit exasperated wheeling the ECG machine around her elevated legs while she massaged her neck. She insisted on remaining at her post, however, and the continuing comments from patients about her loyalty and spunk began to grate.

But youth is resilient. Within three days her feet were down, and my mood was up and the office a Bengay-free zone.

On Thursday afternoon of the following week, Sue Alice asked if she could leave a little early. It was her anniversary, and she was planning a cookout for her husband. Though I'd have preferred more notice, I relented and wished her a pleasant time.

I was off that evening, so the phone call from the ER doctor was unexpected.

"Do you want to treat this burn, or shall I?" he asked.

"What burn?"

"Your nurse. Left forearm, mostly first and some second-degree. Something about lighting a grill."

On Friday morning her left arm was bandaged and slung (yes, she was left-handed), and last week's ankle Bengayed and Ace-wrapped again ("jumping back from the explosion"). With Sue Alice back on the disabled list, my secretary assumed some nursing duties, and we managed to get through the days until Sue Alice returned.

After three months on the job, she developed an allergy to the media used in urine cultures. That's when I sat her down for an in-depth review of her succession of maladies. I indicated that fate can certainly be unkind, and although I wished to be fair, an office schedule had to be maintained. We discussed good work habits at length, and shortly thereafter things improved. Sort of.

Over the next four weeks I treated her for an episode of gastroenteritis, a urinary tract infection, and a bout of oral candidiasis. The mask she wore when using the incubator wasn't as disconcerting as the sunglasses and tennis visor she affected on her "migraine" days. At least she was functioning, so I was thankful. Though some patients seemed unnerved by her appearance, none made any comments to me. During this period her husband, a diabetic, also became a patient.

Solicitously, I suggested a neurologist for her recurring headaches. Little did I suspect this would evolve into three office visits, two EEGs, a CT scan, a biofeedback interlude, and a series of psychological interviews. A side effect of the medication she was prescribed was tardive dyskinesia, an involuntary smacking of the lips. Between the tennis visor, sunglasses, cervical brace, and her mouth suddenly taking on a life of its own, she was a sight to behold.

The neurological workup was accomplished largely during office hours. We again discussed the situation in some detail. The talk concluded with a request for time to visit her terminally ill aunt in Philadelphia. She realized the difficulties she was causing, but if I could just bear with her...

I continued to do so, but the last straw was when Gestalt died. That was Sue Alice's dog. After the cremation and normal grief period, she returned to the office and announced that she and her husband had replaced Gestalt with Angst, a puppy. Alas, Angst soon aspirated a bone and underwent emergency surgery. When his recovery cost me Sue Alice's services for three days, my resolve hardened. She had to go.

The problem was, despite the absences and aggravations, I had no evidence of any incompetence or dishonesty. Only recently had I begun keeping track of her time away from the office. Legally I felt insecure in firing her.

Sue Alice made it easy. A pharmacist called to question a prescription for Fiorinal with Codeine.

"The signature looks okay," he said, "but not the rest of the script."

"Can you describe the customer?"

"Sure. Thin girl, long ponytail, cervical brace."

Our confrontation was brief. She admitted forging the prescription, and we agreed that she should leave. I offered to make arrangements for follow-up counseling. She and the Bengay aroma left my office.

During her six months with me, Sue Alice had worked just over three; I seldom got a full week out of her. A lesson had been learned: be wary of flowery references short on specifics, establish and adhere to a sick time and vacation policy, and be wary of applicants who carry their own Kleenex.

A few months later, Sue Alice's aunt from Philadelphia —the one with the terminal illness – dropped in for a tetanus shot prior to a trip to Africa.

"How's Sue Alice doing?" I asked.

"Not working right now," she answered. "Staying home with Angst, the poor thing. He's got sugar diabetes too."

The Con

Drug seekers are a concern in any medical practice. Certainly they were in mine. Some are easily recognized: anxious, distraught, disheveled "frequent flyers" presenting with the lamest of excuses for their narcotic needs. In fact, some will admit straight out what they want: "just a few until I can see my own doc." Others seek narcotics not for their own use but to sell to others. A very lucrative business and an enviable lifestyle can be acquired in this fashion.

Then there are the more nuanced presentations: lost prescriptions, own doctor not available, recent injury, back pain with blood in urine, and the list continues. Part of the problem: pain is difficult to quantify. Its presence can't be proven by x-ray or blood tests; severe pain can co-exist with a negative physical examination. In the end it comes down to the patient's story – does it sound reasonable? —and what your eyes see, hands feel, and gut tells you.

Over the years I had developed an unscientific, biased profile for those I call the "uptown drug seekers." Their age ranged from mid-thirties through late-forties, and they presented as well-dressed businessmen, albeit a little rough around the edges – frayed shirt collar, scuffed shoes, worn jacket – but articulate, personable, with a clean appearance. Almost always they had a cane.

What set them apart was their deference. As soon as you entered the exam room, they stood and took a few steps toward you – introducing their limp – and offered a moist palm and tentative handshake.

"Good morning, Sir. Sorry to bother you on such a busy morning. I won't take much of your time. A pharmacist recommended you, said you were the best in town."

With some variations, that started the typical conversation. With the trifecta of cane, limp, and exaggerated courtesy, a red flag fluttered – although I did like the part about being "the best in town."

Such a patient presented in my office one summer morning seeking a prescription refill. He is recalled because he was more imaginative than most.

Alec (name altered) was forty-one years old and had arrived in the area a week earlier to visit an ailing relative. Unfortunately, the person died, and it was necessary for him to stay to help settle the estate.

"You know how these things are, Doctor." His tone was conspiratorial. "You fellows deal with death all the time. God bless you."

"So what can I do for you today, Alec?" I asked.

"Well, his death threw off my plans, messed up my med schedule. I've run out of my back pills. The pharmacist told me he can't accept narcotic prescriptions from out-of-state over the phone. I'm alright now but the weekend's coming."

"What do you take?"

"Percocet."

"Do you have a pill bottle, so I can see what you're taking, the strength, how many you were prescribed, things like that? It would help."

"No, I don't. I take whatever it says on my discharge summary."

"What discharge summary?"

Sweat was forming on his forehead. He wiped it with a hand-kerchief. "I know you have to be careful about giving out drugs these days, so I brought a copy of my last discharge from San Francisco General so you can read for yourself."

The document was three pages long, each displaying the hospital letterhead. Alec's past history was impressive, with multiple back procedures over a five-year period. Medications taken on a regular basis included Percocet.

"It's all there, Doc, for your reading pleasure," he said, smiling. "I can show you the scars if you like." His eyes were expectant and friendly.

"Let me take it into my office and look it over. I'll be back."

I scanned the document. Nothing was amiss. But something didn't ring true. My trifecta profile had seldom been wrong. In spite of the time differential, I decided to call the hospital; maybe someone would be in medical records.

There was, and she checked admissions over the past year and could find no name that matched the name on the discharge papers. Checking the hospital number on the summary, however, produced another name. The lady said she couldn't understand that but would get to the bottom of it and call me back.

I returned to Alec and told him what I had done and that there was no record of his admission. He took the news calmly, and to his credit, remained as pleasant and courteous as ever. "There must be some mistake," he offered. "Some mix-up. I'll call out there and straighten it out." His dismay seemed sincere. He thanked me for my help, and after a good-bye to both secretary and nurse, he was on his way.

San Francisco General did get back to me. Someone in medical records remembered Alec's last name. It turned out that his wife worked in their department as a transcriptionist. She had chosen a discharge summary which best fit her husband's profile and drug needs, and inserted his name.

Though I felt quite self-righteous and clever, having recognized and thwarted the scam, there was also a twinge of admiration for the ingenuity involved on Alec's part.

The disquieting thought in these scenarios: addiction doesn't confer an immunity to pain or the possibility of other issues. This particular incident was quite straight forward, but assuming every request for medication in this population is bogus has led to unfortunate conclusions.

The Mob Connection

One summer morning in 1984, my secretary informed me, "A lawyer is on the phone and wishes to speak with you."

He introduced himself. His name was familiar as one of the top defense attorneys in Rhode Island.

"Doctor, I'm calling you because I understand you are a flight surgeon with the National Guard."

"That's correct."

"I have a client who has been ordered to appear in Florida for trial. It is my contention, and that of his cardiologist, that his medical condition precludes air travel. I would like you to review his medical records and give your opinion."

"But his cardiologist already has."

"Yes, he will be my primary witness. But to reinforce his opinion I'd like to have a doctor available who has a background in aviation medicine. Would you be able to do that for us? The hearing is next week."

"Sure, I don't see why not."

"That's great." He identified his client, a man associated with organized crime in New England.

I asked if that was the case.

I heard a chuckle at the other end of the line. "Yes, but you can't back out now." His tone was joking.

A copy of the gentleman's (whom I nicknamed The Don), voluminous record was dropped off at the office. I spent part of the weekend reviewing it. A pattern of cardiac and pulmonary difficulties became obvious. Since the air pressure in a plane cabin is relatively low compared to sea level, less oxygen is taken up by the blood, which can further stress an already compromised breathing system.

The attorney called Monday morning. "Did you have a chance to read the reports, Doctor?"

"I did."

"And ...?"

"The flight could jeopardize your client's health status."

"That's excellent. He will be pleased."

The court day arrived. I was present in my Air Force uniform – at the request of the defense team. During the course of testimony, I learned that their client had been deemed medically unfit to travel three years earlier. The Rhode Island Hospital cardiologist testified that on the basis of his recent physical examination, his status had not improved. The judge once again ruled that air travel constituted a medical risk for The Don. I wasn't called upon for my input.

Watching the proceedings, I was struck by the disparity between the opposing legal camps. The State was represented by three lawyers – two with crew cuts – trim, eager, brisk in their walk, articulate in their presentation, and who seemed proficient, but obviously, the ink on their law degree had only recently dried.

The defense, relaxed but attentive, was ancient in comparison. Attired in dark, bespoke suits; available hair tinged gray; Ben Franklin glasses astride weathered faces; portly evidence of lives well lived, they exuded expertise and experience.

The perception was of an unfair match-up: the big leagues against a farm team, superior court versus a traffic tribunal. It highlighted – for me at least – how obviously the scales of justice were tilted toward those who could afford superior representation.

Three weeks later, my secretary mentioned that the bill for my services on behalf of The Don had not been paid, about $300 as I recollect. With a smile, I suggested she give him a call and threaten him with collection agency action if he didn't pay up. She demurred, saying that since he was *my* friend, that could be *my* task.

Sometime later the check arrived. An accompanying, hand-written note thanked me for my help.

A few days before Thanksgiving, while chatting in the waiting room with a patient's relative, the door opened and two heavyset men walked in. Each wore a dark coat and soft hat, and between them they carried a large, old-fashioned laundry basket. It contained a turkey, various vegetables, Italian bread, and three bottles of wine. They placed it on the floor in front of me. The heavier one announced, "Dis is from da boss." The other man smiled, nodded, and tipped his hat to an astonished secretary. Then they turned and left.

It was a perfect scene, right out of Hollywood casting. Francis Ford Coppola would have been proud. And the turkey wasn't bad, either.

Young Guns Settle In

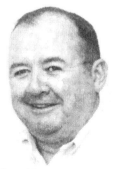

William McDermott, M.D.
South County Hospital

The Pediatrician

By the early 1970s, Dr. William McDermott had cornered the pediatric market. The central factor in his improved practice numbers related to his expertise and experience, but also to the growing youngster population (South County increasingly a bedroom community of Providence), the attrition of older physicians, and the influx of internists who did not deal with kids.

A treat at medical staff meetings was witnessing Dr. McDermott's bombast, in the form of monthly eruptions railing against any number of issues, but particularly government's intrusion into medical care. The assembled, many in sympathy – knowing Bill was merely acting out, blowing off steam after four weeks of dealing with crying babies and concerned mothers – not only tolerated it but egged him on. Spirited exchanges ensued. Then, his position made clear, chest unburdened, catharsis achieved, a more relaxed Bill resumed his seat, smile lines creasing his Irish features.

Dr. McDermott – along with Roger Ashley, MD, who joined his practice – treated our five children until their teenage years without charge, a professional courtesy extended to physicians' families by most offices at that time.

The Surgeon

Dr. Robert Conrad's surgical numbers rose steadily, and by the mid-1970s, he had an established practice. With a direct, often brusque style, he served the hospital well in various capacities but most specifically as chief of emergency services, a post he occupied for most of the decade. In 1978, through a program at Rhode Island College (RIC), Dr. Conrad trained and brought the first Emergency Medical Technicians (EMTs) to the South County area.

Bob's decision spectrum had few shades of gray. Situations were viewed as black or white; he was either all in or all out. He was not shy in promoting his projects or hesitant to employ a few bells and whistles if that would hasten the outcome. He successfully lobbied for an expanded emergency department which became operational in 1976, and after a fishing boat disaster, when rapid transport to a tertiary hospital wasn't available, his efforts led to the construction of a heliport at SCH, the first Rhode Island hospital to have this capability.

Implementing a physician rotation to Block Island to cover that community when the island was without a physician, was another goal accomplished. Three or four of us worked five day segments, usually during the winter months, until the vacancy had been filled. Accommodations were provided, and although the winter season was harsh, we got a sense of what island living was all about – the isolation, the untrammeled beauty of the place, the tight community – the only downside being that everyone on the island knew where you were. There was no escape.

Dr. Conrad owned an island on the Great Salt Pond where, during the summer months, he raised a variety of animals: sheep, turkeys, pigs, and guinea hens. The pigs were enclosed in a pen, the others roamed free. At the end of the season, the group (fattened by four months of easy living), was transported to the mainland and the farm and slaughterhouse of Spud Mack.

One day, Spud mentioned to Dr. Conrad that one of his cows was ill: he was concerned that the animal had swallowed a piece of metal while chomping for food.

After some consideration, Bob came up with a plan to rule out the possibility: transport the cow to the back of the hospital, wheel out the portable x-ray machine, snap a picture, and the answer would be readily apparent.

But as is often the case with good intentions, things can go amiss. The portable machine did not have the capacity to penetrate the considerable girth of the patient. Thwarted, but not to be denied, Bob pressed on. A bed sheet was thrown over the cow to camouflage her cautious entrance into the hospital and the nearby radiology department. That the enormity of a several hundred-pound animal would somehow be diminished by a bed sheet seemed almost reasonable in this Marx Brothers scenario. The entourage – Spud, Bob, two technicians, and the cow – continued to x-ray, only to be halted by the bewildered bovine's immense evacuation.

Responding quickly, Dr. Conrad grabbed a couple of x-ray folders and scooped the viscous mound into a waste basket. Suddenly, a pair of white shoes came into his view. He looked up to see a nurse supervisor with a puzzled look on her face.

"What are you doing, Dr. Conrad?"

"Cleaning up cow shit. What does it look like I'm doing?"

"What cow?"

"That one." He pointed toward the x-ray room. Filling the observation window was a broad, brown-spackled backside and a tail rhythmically swinging.

"Get that thing out of here," she said, her voice rising. "Now!"

The x-ray was taken. Spud and the cow retraced their steps back to the truck, avoiding the large stain on the carpet.

Knowing Mr. Ford would hear about the incident, Bob (in a preemptive move), arranged an appointment for the following morning.

The meeting was brief. Dr. Conrad's attempt at humor: "It's a community hospital, Mr. Ford, our doors are open to all. No discrimination around here," was met with a dismissive stare.

"Don't let it happen again, Dr. Conrad," was Mr. Ford's only contribution to the conversation.

The results of the saga were mixed: no metal was detected in the abdomen, though the cow died a short time later, a virus suspected. Dr. Conrad and the tale of the cow became firmly fixed in the lore and legend of South County Hospital.

However, the most controversial case of Dr. Conrad's career, one with profound moral, ethical, and legal implications, happened in 1988. It concerned Marcia Gray, a forty-nine-year-old lady who in 1986 suffered a cerebral hemorrhage that left her in a persistent vegetative state. After four unsuccessful surgeries, she was admitted to the state general hospital, where she remained for two years. Her family went to court to fight for her right to die, and on October 17, 1988, a U.S. district judge ordered her feeding tube removed.

The general hospital refused to comply with the federal order, as did other institutions. Their concern: the legal implications of a procedure which effectively resulted in the death of a patient.

Dr. Conrad, with the approval of the hospital's board of trustees, arranged the transfer of the patient to South County Hospital. During the transport, Dr. Conrad removed the feeding tube. Two weeks after her admission, Marcia Gray passed away. The implications of the decision still resonate in the legal community. The consensus of opinion, both secular and religious, was overwhelmingly in favor of Bob's intervention.

The Obstetrician/Gynecologist

As fewer primary care practitioners became involved in obstetrics, Dr. Joseph O'Neill became the only show in town. The days of the office phone that seldom rang were long gone. He was spending more time in the hospital than at home and two- to three-day stretches there were not unusual. Joseph maintained that pace for seven years at which time his brother, Robert, also board-certified in OB/GYN and stationed at the Quonset Point Naval Hospital, provided part-time relief.

Although likely unaware of it at the time, Joseph was the key player, both symbolically and in fact, in the changing of the hospital guard.

The medical staff officer positions – president, vice president, secretary, and treasurer – were filled by older physicians. Dr. Walsh had occupied the top slot since 1967. The other positions were rotated amongst the rest of the group. The ability to maintain these positions for that period of time was dependent on two factors: a plurality which was becoming, in the late 1960s, increasingly thin; and the prerogatives enjoyed by Dr. Walsh as president.

At the annual election staff meeting, when the cohort of elders presented their slate of officers to the president, Dr. Walsh acknowledged their receipt and immediately closed further nominations from the floor. With no contenders, the slate was accepted.

Frustration mounted, and a mini-rebellion among the younger staff was building. Dr. Murdocco, the ENT surgeon who joined the staff in 1972, recalled meetings at his home where plans were hatched to replace the leadership.

The key position to secure was medical staff president, whose authority decided service chiefs, committee chairs, and staff appointments. The choice to lead the coup and capture the presidency came down, fittingly, to two of the young guns: Bob Conrad and Joe O'Neill.

The consensus was that Bob, although certainly able, was too much the brash, outspoken surgeon with a penchant for ruffling feathers. Joe O'Neill, although similarly capable, was viewed as more affable, reasonable, and less likely to incite animosity.

A quiet campaign ensued, but the incumbent ranks remained solid. While they remained united, they could easily thwart any challenges. A crack in their ranks appeared unlikely until one day there was one – in the person of Dr. Attilio Manganaro.

In 1973 the staff gathered in the large conference room for the election and presumably to witness the usual political shenanigans. After Dr. Walsh announced "elections" as the next agenda item, he read off the pre-packaged list of candidates. Before Jack's gavel could sound the close of nominations, Attilio was on his feet offering, in the form of a motion, his slate of candidates for the coming year. Joseph O'Neill was at the top of the ticket. As Dr. Manganaro took his seat, he declared for all to hear, "It's time for a change."

Dr. Walsh appeared flummoxed, taken aback by the turn of events. Here was one of their own, one of the stalwarts, challenging the agreed-upon slate. With little recourse, he allowed the motion and subsequent vote. The old timers ran a distant second. Whether Joe made Dr. Manganaro an offer he couldn't refuse remains conjecture to this day.

Dr. Manganaro wasn't easily forgiven by his colleagues for his defection. Approximately twenty years later, during a beach chat with Dr. Erwin Siegmund, a friend of Dr. Walsh, Erwin became visibly distressed, flipping his cigarette into the surf, when I recalled that election. A discussion followed. His position, after two decades of reflection, could best be summed up with his parting comment: "I'll never forgive that little sonofabitch."

This election signaled the close of an era, the last hurrah for a group who for twenty years had controlled the political agenda of the medical staff. Like farmers in the old west who put up fences to protect their turf from newcomers – the cattlemen and their herds – they lost the battle. The torch had been passed. It should be noted that these same "stubborn, old docs" had for decades provided competent medical care to a grateful community. May the current crop be as successful.

Joe served a second term as president in 1995. In 2001 he became the vice president of medical affairs at the hospital, the unanimous choice of the board of trustees, and more telling, his peers. Joe was responsible for a broad range of activities, including: credentialing of physicians, peer review activities, monitoring the activities of clinical departments, and acting as liaison between the medical staff, administration, and board of trustees.

When his brother Robert finished his stint in the Navy, they formed a practice and for decades ably served the female population of South County. The brothers O'Neill – a class act.

THE HOME FRONT

Whatever Lila Wants...

While all this was going on, the McKee family was pleased to welcome two new members: Sean Patrick on January 28, 1972, whom I was privileged to deliver into the world, and Clare Margaret on May 1, 1973. I think it can be said that Pat and I proved in conclusive fashion the prescience of the lady back at Otis AFB. We did create some beautiful kids.

Our first Rhode Island home on Hillcrest Road became too small for our expanding census. We purchased a dwelling inspired by Harry Mars, a talented Native Indian stone mason, on Dockray Road in Wakefield.

Real estate had interested me for a long time. Exploring raw land and tracking through old houses was my idea of a fun afternoon. My favorite community was Narragansett, and I was always on the lookout for properties there, especially those with a rich history or in reasonable proximity to the ocean. It was on such an excursion that I met Lila Delman.

I attended an auction at Dunmere, a mansion on Ocean Road built originally for the Dun of Dun and Bradstreet fame. Lila, a real estate agent, was in attendance. The magnificent property included thirteen acres on the ocean, a broad sweep of lawn to the sea, and a three-story main house of shingle/stone construction which brought to mind on that drizzly, foggy day, Heathcliff's Wuthering Heights. The gardener's cottage at the entrance, of similar construction and equally imposing, had been converted into a less exuberant living space. The entire package was coming onto the market.

Lila, a formidable presence, moved among and chatted with the few attendees, and in the process, introduced herself to Pat and me. A pleasant chat followed, at the end of which she told me I should buy the place.

"Isn't it gorgeous?" Lila asked.

"Yes, it is," we both agreed.

"It can be yours," she said, "the whole shebang, the thirteen acres, the works, for $250,000."

"Lila," I said, "we just came down to see the place. If you said $20,000 I couldn't do it."

"Do you have any friends?"

"Some, but no one with that kind of money."

"That's too bad," she said. "It's a great buy."

And a great buy it would have been.

Lila, the hardest working real estate agent in my memory, always kept in touch. Any property she felt we might have an interest in she contacted us. And no matter how many no's she received, she never lost her good humor, her last call as enthusiastic as the first. It was just such a call on a spring day some months later that made for a highly unusual showing.

The house was an older Victorian, two blocks from the ocean on Central Street. It needed some work, she added, but was worth taking a look at. Pat and I arranged to meet Lila at her office on Ocean Road.

The office appeared disorganized. Keys to the various properties she was handling hung from hooks on a large board. A circular white tag on each identified the address. But there were also unmarked keys loose on the desk and in the desk drawer she was rummaging through when we arrived. A nearby desk was littered with letters, files, documents, and Post-it notes.

As she bustled about, key now in hand, she explained that the owner of the Central Street property was an older lady who had decided to stay in Florida and sell her place in Narragansett. Lila also mentioned that the house was presently occupied.

When she called to give the renter a "heads-up" that we would be visiting, there was no answer.

"I'm sure it will be fine," she added.

There were two cars in the driveway when we arrived but no response to the doorbell. We walked around the first floor. The house did need some work, but structurally seemed fine.

As I passed the dining room window, I saw what at first appeared to be a large, black whale beached in the side yard. It was an oil tank, covered with slabs of grass and dirt.

Lila had no quick answer for this apparition, shrugging it off as a minor problem, as though it happened with houses all the time. Her explanation: the tank was likely empty and "all the rain we had this spring probably floated it up." Pat wondered if it happened every year. Lila didn't know but assured us she'd speak to the owner and have it taken care of.

On the second floor were three bedrooms. We walked through two of them. The door to the third was closed. When Lila knocked on the door, a female voice answered. "Who's that?"

"Lila, the real estate lady. I'm showing the house."

"Come back later," the voice said. "I'm taking a nap."

What the person in the bedroom didn't know was that when Lila made up her mind to show a house, that house was going to be shown.

"It will only take a minute."

Lila opened the door. A young couple were in bed. The man dived under the sheets, covering his head with a pillow. The woman sat up, holding a blanket to her chest. "Please leave," she demanded.

"In a minute, Dear," Lila answered.

Without a hint of awkwardness, Lila started to talk about central heating. Pat and I edged toward the door.

"And this is the bathroom," said Lila. She pushed open the door. "Well, look at this."

We went over. There in the tub, in about six inches of water, was a small alligator.

"What's his name?" asked Lila.

"I don't know," said the young woman. "Please leave."

We did. Lila's closing comment: "Have a good day, you two."

We didn't buy the house. But a few years later, it became the residence of Claudine Schneider, Rhode Island's congressional representative. An invite to a wedding reception brought us back to the place a few years later. Ms. Schneider had done a great restoration job. I asked her if there had been any whale or alligator sightings. She seemed confused. I didn't bother explaining.

Grandmother Dalton

An additional benefit of our move to Rhode Island: it allowed Pat's mother Julia, a widow and nursery nurse at Boston City Hospital, to visit more frequently. Always a welcome presence in our household – none of the negative mother-in-law aspersions applied. She was particularly indispensable to our family following the addition of Clare (who had a fragile post-natal course).

My relationship with Pat had been well underway before Mrs. Dalton and I had our first meeting. I sensed her acceptance of Pat's choice of male company didn't automatically include her approval. In spite of my boyish charm and other endearing qualities, she was wary of my intentions, with some justification.

One day, some months later, in a joking manner, I said, "I'll soon be taking Pat off your hands," (implying a considerable sacrifice on my part). Her smiling Irish eyes, present to that point, vanished without a trace.

"I beg your pardon," she replied, "but I think you've got it wrong. You're certainly not doing me any favors, and," she paused for a sip of water, "I have my doubts you're doing my daughter any either."

My insistence that I was just joking did not rescue either me or the remainder of a frosty conversation. Behind her quiet demeanor and amiable manner, there lurked a tiger; you didn't mess with Julia Dalton when it came to her cubs.

Grandma Dalton and I eventually became good friends. A mutual respect and affection evolved. And beyond that, she was my advocate when an ally was needed, the voice of calm and reason when occasionally that was in short supply.

Her visits always included small gifts for the children which the older ones remember to this day. She enjoyed the South County area and was more than willing to forsake the traffic and congestion of Boston to move here. Plans had progressed to the extent that in August of 1973 she had taken an apartment on Main St. in Wakefield, awaiting her retirement date in approximately one month. The paperwork had been completed.

Pat and I had made plans to attend a weekend medical conference in Montreal. Grandma Dalton was to stay with the kids; Matt and I went to pick her up. Seconds after entering her apartment he rushed out. "Grandma's on the floor!" Matt stayed in the car while I went in. There were no signs of life. Five packages, neatly wrapped, were on the table next to her. She was sixty-four years old.

Summer Cottage

The eventual move to Narragansett came about in serendipitous fashion. At the time, I was the physician for the community of nuns who taught at Monsignor Clarke School, a K-8 Catholic school in town. They lived at La Sata, a large dwelling on Central Street in Narragansett, formerly owned by "Black Jack" Bouvier, uncle of Jackie Kennedy. Jackie reportedly spent considerable time there as a young girl.

Making small talk with Sister Constance at the end of her visit, I casually asked if there were any properties for sale in her neighborhood. She didn't know of any but mentioned that the house next to theirs, 106 Central Street, might be available soon. Sister explained that she frequently spent time as a companion to the owner, Mrs. Harrah, an elderly lady who lived there alone during the summer months. During their chats, Mrs. Harrah had occasionally mentioned the size of the house and her advancing age, intimating she might consider selling the property. "You should take a look at it," Sister added. "It would be a great place to bring up kids."

My interest piqued, Sister Constance agreed to speak with Mrs. Harrah's son Eric, a lawyer, as to the possibility of walking through the place.

After work, I drove past the house: a three-story, hip-roofed Victorian situated on a nicely landscaped parcel of land. Stone pillars marked the two entrances to a circular drive, a broad porch extended around the front of the house. At first glance its size seemed overwhelming, but I liked the look, the home's name (Sunnymead) engraved on the pillars and its location.

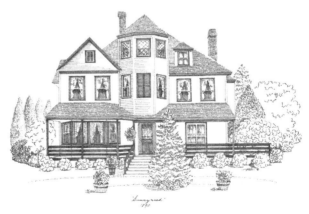

Pencil sketch of Sunnymead, Central Street, Narragansett

That night I mentioned to Pat that I had a place to show her the following day. Her reactions were similar to mine, but she seemed interested. "It would be fun to walk around the house, if nothing else," was her comment as we drove away.

Within days, Eric Harrah contacted me, and an appointment was made to tour the residence.

It was an impressive twenty-seven room layout. The four bedrooms on the second floor each had a fireplace, bathroom and marble vanity. The third floor, formerly the servant's quarters, also had four bedrooms and a bathroom. Most of the first floor was taken up with the living room, a dining room with stained glass windows, and library (each with a fireplace, wainscoting and parquet oak floors). In the rear portion was the kitchen. Two adjoining rooms and a bathroom were described by Eric, though not shown because they hadn't been used for many years. He also reported a small apartment in the three-car garage.

We expressed our interest in the property. Eric said he would set up a time for us to meet his mother and the family.

In the interim I contacted Winifred Kissouth, a patient of mine and the town's unofficial historian. I told her we were looking at a house on Central Street for possible purchase.

"Sister Constance mentioned it has an interesting history, and I wondered if you wouldn't mind doing some research for me?"

"I know the property well, Dr. McKee," Mrs. Kissouth said. "A few years ago, it was included in my project on Central Street homes."

Her findings: Built in 1890 as a summer cottage, Sunnymead was owned by the three Gwynn sisters, remnants of a wealthy Philadelphia family. The oldest of the three, Alice, had married Cornelius Vanderbilt II, grandson of the self-proclaimed commodore. A reception celebrating their union was held at Sunnymead. One of the remaining sisters, Cetti, married William Shepherd; they had a daughter, Maude – the present occupant – who married a man named Harrah. After his death Maude lived in the house by herself, although her daughter was across the street and her son next door.

On the day of our appointment, a well-tended, gray-haired lady wearing pink slippers received us in the first floor sitting room. A green shawl was drawn about her shoulders. A delicately poised hand was offered to each of us. Mrs. Harrah suggested we sit in the two straight-back chairs arranged in front of her. Tea was offered, but we declined. Also present was Eric, her daughter Lorna, and son-in-law Jay.

General conversation followed, touching on the housing market, something of our background, a synopsis of our children's activities, people she or the others knew with whom we might be familiar, vacation locations that might have been mutually enjoyed. I had the impression that she was searching for something in our pedigree that would complement hers. Perhaps an uncle who was a Wall Street broker, a grandparent who went to Yale, a niece who married an obscure Austrian count: some credential of affluence or celebrity that she could relay to friends to assure their family home (since 1891), was sold to the right "type." If she was disappointed with our pedestrian background, she didn't let on.

Mrs. Harrah was a charming lady. Her reminiscences were delightful. She recalled with remarkable clarity, the rich tapestry of life in a house which seemed in the telling always filled with "interesting" people. And especially remembered were "the wonderful parties" during Prohibition days, when guests were fortified with the offerings of Billy McCoy.

> **Historical aside:** *In 1920 the 18th amendment to the Constitution (which Rhode Island – and Connecticut never ratified), became the law of the land. The amendment essentially prohibited the manufacture, distribution, and sale of alcohol—notably not its consumption or private possession.*
>
> *Rhode Island's disapproval stemmed from the economic benefits alcohol had brought to the state. In post-revolutionary war days (until Moses Brown and Samuel Slater initiated the Industrial Revolution with their mill on the Blackstone River in Pawtucket), the state's economy was sustained in*

large measure by the sale of alcohol, primarily rum. Scores of distilleries – thirty-seven in Providence alone – were scattered throughout Rhode Island. A robust market developed (exceeding a million gallons annually), encompassing the north eastern section of the country and as far south as the Carolinas.

With the sympathies of the populace and the legislature thus known–and with 400 miles of coast-line–Rhode Island became a major player in the bootlegging industry.

Of the rum runners on Narragansett Bay, Bill McCoy was legendary. A boutique bootlegger–never connected with the crime syndicates – he dealt with only quality products – Cutty Sack, Gordons, guaranteed free of adulterants and diluents, the "real McCoy."

Locally, a favored off-loading site for the booze was the small cove at the northern end of Scarborough Beach. A narrow path led to Ocean Road where trucks waited. Deliveries were made at the ocean-front mansions and hotels in town. The Ocean Rose Inn –with gambling on the second floor and "comfort rooms" on the third– was a regular customer. Bill McCoy – who didn't drink – was said to have a girlfriend there whom he visited when delivering to this section of the coast.

Mrs. Harrah recalled polo and golfing days at Point Judith Country Club, big bands that played the casino, and Lester Lanin's Society Orchestra at the Dunes Club. During that era, Narragansett defined East Coast summer society, and Newport was just an aspiring newcomer. "We sent them the people we didn't want here," Mrs. Harrah said, smiling.

It was a wonderful conversation, one which I was sorry to see end. "If we reach an arrangement," Mrs. Harrah said, "you'd be the first owners outside the family." Money was not discussed. Eric would be in touch.

The meeting with Eric was brief. The asking price was $55,000. I offered $45,000. We settled for $50,000. Pat and I still hadn't walked through the entire house yet.

Then we did. Noted were: a warren of rooms in disrepair, uneven floors warped by moisture, exposed water pipes in the kitchen, no insulation, and no heating system. Much of this we knew, but ownership sharpens the reality. The large rooms on the first floor and the bedrooms on the second had only shallow fireplaces, designed to remove the chill of a cool summer day. Many of the large, drafty windows refused to open.

Misgivings briefly surfaced.

But slowly we chipped away at the deficiencies until it became a warm, livable home, and as Sister Constance had suggested, a great place to bring up kids. Maintaining the tradition Mrs. Harrah spoke of, we threw some great parties, especially during Christmas season, even though the drinks lacked the frisson of bootlegged hooch.

In retrospect, the purchase of this ark of a house was one of the most impractical, poorly thought out, unrealistic, best decisions of my life. It was a wonderful home for thirty-five years, our shelter through storms, our delight during sunny times, and now our fond memory.

Family Matters

At home, all was well, the kids healthy and getting taller every week. Matthew was enrolled at Bishop Hendricken High School in Warwick, while Ellen, Kate, and Sean were at Monseigneur Clarke in Narragansett. Clare was in the first grade program at Wakefield Elementary School.

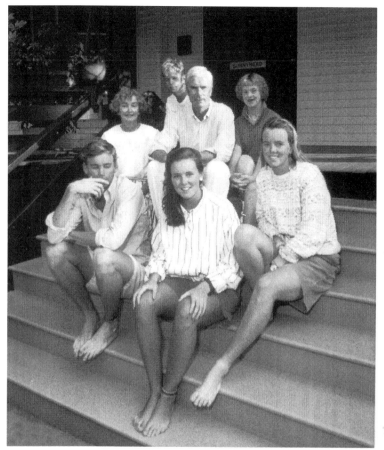

On steps of Sunnymead, from left to right: Matthew, Pat, Sean, the author, Ellen, Clare, and Kate

Believing that peer pressure was a key determinant of teenage behavior, Pat and I felt that sports, and the kids who played them, offered a healthy diversion for restless minds and bodies, at least for a few hours each week. In our group, swimming was the favored activity and not a hard sell. All competed at various levels, and friendships made in the pool continue to this day.

In the family recreational area, everyone skied, though no one competitively except Clare. For many years, during December and February vacations, our tribe headed north, particularly enjoying Waterville Valley. There are few sports which have the entire family enjoying the same activity at the same time, and skiing is one of them. Hunkered down with the brood in the evening, wind howling off the mountain, re-skiing the day, a couple of beers for good old Dad, a game of cards, often a movie – were some of the best times for the McKee family.

An Accomplishment of Sorts

As a youth, I'd spent large chunks of my summers caddying at the Point Judith Country Club. That was my choice, an escape from the never-ending chores at home: cutting and raking grass, tending flower gardens, weeding a large vegetable garden – the list went on. I enjoyed caddying and was good at it. I was also proud to bring home and display my earnings, flipping the five or six dollars on the kitchen table for all to see, gambler style, and then modestly accepting compliments. "Look how much Gene made today, Grandma," my aunt would say. Of course, I never saw the money again. "Put away for college."

Since the family cottage in Point Judith was remote from other homes, there was no one my age to play with. The golf course filled that void. Kids from Wakefield and Peace Dale, predominantly black, turned up daily. The main activities, when not on the course, were fighting; playing card games; exploring the old polo barns and climbing up into the rafters, hoping to find bats and roust them from their perches.

I often announced to my fellow caddies, "One day I'm gonna be a member at the Point Judith Country Club. I'll have my *own* caddy and give him a big tip." They all laughed.

On an early spring morning in the late 1970s, I strode down the first fairway at Point Judith, my adolescent aspirations realized. But as I came to understand over the years, it came at a price: my mental stability.

Golf, it has been said, was invented by a man torn with guilt, eager to atone for his sins. In essence, it's a gentlemanly form of masochism clothed in the guise of camaraderie and forced good humor. From experience, I know this to be true.

For many summers, the golf gods led me along, whetting my appetite, allowing a string of acceptable rounds which lured me to lessons and an array of purchases to include clubs customized to my swing speed, physique, and ability. A single-digit handicap, the ads promised, was just a matter of time. Any number of golf magazines were strewn on my coffee table and bedside stand.

Once securely hooked, a vengeful deity made her move (note gender). First with my putter: balls a foot or two from the pin, tap-ins, lipped the cup or, deflected by an untended ball mark, skipped by the hole. Then, one by one, the other clubs, formerly seamless extensions of my arms, transformed into clumsy strangers in my frequently changing grip. Even my trusted driver failed me. Duck hooks, embarrassing slices, unmentionable shanks were commonplace. Strong consideration was given to the possibility of a developing neurological condition.

This scenario, with minor alterations, continued for a number of seasons. Beautiful summer days were ruined. Winter ones were also affected. Memories of heroic golf outings could make weeks of snow and bitter cold more tolerable, but none were available to me.

Two things helped me live with my condition. First, I was not alone. Any honest golfer (an oxymoron some would contend), will admit, after a couple of drinks, to similar tribulations. With appropriate medication, many have survived and continue to play with a measure of success. The second: the wisdom of an older, grizzled caddy.

"Doc," he said, "lower your expectations. Relax. Take what you can get. You ain't never going to be the player you want to be. Shit, no golfer is." He smiled and spit out a chaw of tobacco. "Golf's a lot like sex. You can still enjoy it even though you ain't no good at it."

The Isle of Saints and Sinners

In the early spring of 1981, while leafing through a medical publication, I came across an advertisement offering a cottage for rent on the west coast of Ireland for a period of either two weeks or the entire summer. It was located in the town of Inch on the Dingle Peninsula and offered a "panoramic view of the bay. All amenities provided." That stimulus, combined with my inordinate nostalgia for the auld sod and the wish that our children be introduced to the land of their ancestors, prompted – after some discussion – unanimous approval for the trip. The plan was to make Inch our home base and take day trips to explore the surrounding areas.

Shortly after our arrival, violent weather and a dismal forecast, mildewed accommodations, and the smell of leaking gas, forced a change in plans. The decision was made to leave Inch and bed-and-breakfast our way around the country. There would be no specific itinerary. Comfortably adventurous in an orange VW van (named Whizzer), the officers and crew (ages 15, 12, 11 and 9) set off.

Before departing, we explored the local area and walked the spectacular strand at Inch, a three-mile stretch of clean sand along the curve of Brandon Bay, where St. Brendan the Navigator purportedly launched, by way of Iceland and Greenland, his trip to America. The beach and surrounding locale figured prominently in the 1969 filming of *Ryan's Daughter*, starring Robert Mitchum.

Our wanderings took us through Killarney, the Ring of Kerry, down to Macroom and Ballyvourney in County Cork (home to some of Pat's clan), along the east coast to Youghal, and an overnight stay in a farmhouse which once housed Ryan O'Neal. On to Tralee, Tramore, and Waterford. Lodgings were randomly selected. When the group felt – with the occasional veto by the captain – that it was time to call it a day, we found a bed and breakfast, and that became our home for the night. Each stop was a new experience. The kids loved it.

In Waterford we toured the factory where some of the world's finest crystal creations were conceived and created. The glass, we learned, was a mix of silica, pot ash, and predominantly, lead, the high content of which was responsible for the signature color.

The origin of the crystal production in Waterford dates back to 1783; within a decade the company had established a worldwide reputation. The factory was forced to close in 1851, a casualty of Ireland's potato famine. When it reopened in 1947, artisans from Germany and Switzerland were brought over, as skilled crystal workers were no longer available in Ireland. At the time of our tour, visitors could mix with the glass blowers and the crystal cutters, who were delighted to demonstrate their craft to the kids.

Our arrival in Dun Laoghaire, a village south of Dublin and a port of call in the rape-pillage-and-burn heyday of the Vikings, coincided with Bloomsday, June 16th, the day immortalized in James Joyce's *Ulysses*. That date was chosen by Joyce to commemorate the first encounter with Nora Barnacle, his future wife. With the kids safely tucked into downy beds, Pat and I had a late supper at the Nora Barnacle restaurant. The walls of the establishment were covered with Joyce memorabilia, and the patrons – "students, sophists, and sophisticates"—in various stages of inebriation, were in loud celebration of the great man. Many dressed as Joyce and Nora lookalikes. Everyone was in great form. Jimmy would have been proud.

The following day we explored Dublin where I'd attended medical school at the Royal College of Surgeons. This allowed me to bore my captive audience with my exploits in that fair city, twenty-plus years earlier. Grafton Street – now a vehicle-free thoroughfare – was bustling. The luxuriant aroma of Bewley's coffee shop was unchanged. At Davy Byrnes's pub, not quite as posh as I remember, a pint of Guiness was raised in memory of the foolhardy plots hatched there. The Toby Jug, another old haunt, was gone.

The College of Surgeons was in the process of expansion. St. Stephen's Green, across the street, was in springtime bloom. We visited the Newman Chapel where the children lit candles to ensure continued safety on our trip. The National Library on Kildare Street and its solemn reading room was as I remembered, down to the green-shaded banker lights at each table.

We finished the excursion with tea and finger sandwiches at the Shelbourne Hotel. The atmosphere was that of a drawing room: the discrete hum of conversation from the half-dozen occupied tables now and again ruffled by a soft laugh or the clink of silverware. Even our kids were whispering. A harpist played at the far end of the room, nicely complementing the elegance of the setting.

The next day, our last in Dublin, we took a bus tour into the Boyne Valley, to Tara, Newgrange, and Drogheda. The history of each place was presented in an entertaining fashion by the knowledgeable guide. Our dinner that night was less enriching – fries and burgers at a McDonalds. Clearly, the captain and his co-pilot were outvoted.

The final leg of our journey brought us through the midlands, heading west toward Limerick and Shannon Airport. Our last overnight was at a farm in Ennis, County Clare, where our host showed the kids how to milk a cow. Their attempts were too tentative to produce even a squirt.

Departure day was bright, the sky blue. We settled into our Boston-bound 707, and soon the green of Eire was unfolding on either side of the plane. As we crossed Ireland's west coast, the kids craned their necks, attempting to locate the Dingle Peninsula and the beach at Inch. Kate was convinced she saw not only the strand but also our little white cottage.

A glass of red wine in hand, the blue of the Atlantic stretched before me, I looked back on our family adventure. Although hectic and exhausting, it was an interlude in the life of our family that is remembered as clearly – and perhaps more fondly – today as it was thirty-five years ago. The kids were uncomplaining and considerate, courteous and conversant with those they met, and acclimated well in unfamiliar circumstances – all traits of a good traveler. My only regret: not having Clare with us, a little young for the adventure we thought. We'd have her along on the next one.

In 1984 we took another overseas trip, this time with the whole family. In a fashion similar to Ireland – bed and breakfasts, VW van – we spent two weeks visiting Germany, Austria, Switzerland, and France.

I kept a journal for each vacation, the narratives interspersed with photos. I've often said that if the house were burning down, the only things I'd really want to save are the recollections of those two trips.

Passages

In 1981 my father died of heart failure secondary to his pulmonary disease. A long history of smoking was the major contributor. He was eighty-two years old. Visits to a doctor over his lifetime were infrequent, and no medications were taken on a regular basis. When he and my aunt (his sister) moved from Pawtucket to live full time in Narragansett, he had established a relationship with Dr. Nestor, an excellent general practitioner in Wakefield.

My father's life was not noteworthy by the usual standards. No front-page achievements, no prestigious degrees or honors, subject as we all are to fates which sometimes are kind and other times not so much.

He was the most religious person I've ever known, someone who found solace in a faith he never questioned. As a young man, he had aspirations for the priesthood and spent two years at the LaSalette Seminary in R.I. before leaving the order.

While working at the Weybosset Pure Food Market in Providence, he met my mother. A short-lived marriage and my birth followed in rapid succession. Perhaps because of the mores of the time or the dictates of Rome, they never divorced, and to my knowledge, he never had another relationship with a woman. This left a lonely man, the circumstance I most remember about my dad.

He loved to play the horses and travel. On his days off during race season he was a regular at Narragansett Park in Pawtucket. Each year for one week of his two-week vacation, he took a Greyhound to Florida and Hialeah Park. Slow horses and muddy tracks limited his winnings, but the atmosphere and excitement of the racecourse – the lure of the daily double – always brought him back.

A sentimental man, Kate Smith singing "God Bless America" or the grandeur and pomp of a religious ceremony brought him to tears. He was proud of me, so I was told by others, as declarations of that sort didn't trip off his tongue easily.

When I was in medical school in Ireland, he came over by ocean liner to visit for two weeks. For a few days we toured a good portion of the country his father had emigrated from during the famine, then we continued on to England and France. The bed-and-breakfast routine suited him to the ground, along with traveling mostly by auto. For reasons never determined – perhaps the poteen we sampled in Ireland – he came out of his shell, chatting up the families we stayed with, giving them his address, asking to stay in touch. My concerns about his becoming bored or not tolerating the strains of an uncertain itinerary were put to rest.

At the end of the trip, before boarding the tender at Cobh to take him to the waiting liner, my father shook my hand and told me it was his best vacation ever. I was delighted to enhance a man's life, whom I felt had enjoyed so little.

Partners in Aging

In 1977 Pat completed the geriatric nurse practitioner (GNP) curriculum at Boston University and accepted a position at the Wood River Health Center in Hope Valley, thus becoming the first nurse practitioner in Rhode Island.

In 1986, after nine years of ministering to the home-bound elderly in the clinic's rural catchment area, Pat started her own geriatric-care management company, Partners in Aging.

The agency's objective was to address, not just the clinical needs of the patient, but the full spectrum of ancillary issues associated with age and illness: transport to physician visits, insurance issues, medication availability, accessing social services— the list went on.

As with any new endeavor, the challenge was formidable, but Pat, as is typical, seemed to relish the opportunity. She felt that having competent caregivers (the boots on the ground), was the key to a successful program. To this end, mandatory training programs were developed. Registered nurses were hired whose experience best matched the patient cohort; all nurse's aides were certified.

With a reputation for reliability and quality of service already established at Wood River, the transition to the private business model went smoothly. Quite quickly demands for services approached the limits of provider availability, and the company flourished. Within a year, the agency's service area extended from Washington County to Providence and the eastern border of Connecticut.

The success of the company brought both recognition and the interest of other companies providing similar services. Among them was a national group wishing to establish a presence in southern Rhode Island. After protracted discussions, in 1991, Pat agreed to sell the agency. The sales agreement included provisions which stipulated Partners in Aging employees would be kept on in their present positions, without disruption of their insurance coverage.

The transaction was finalized, but their promise to maintain the quality product fell victim to the pull of the bottom line. The new company's attempt to expand the service area didn't include the addition of trained staff necessary for such an endeavor. Patient care suffered as did the morale of the providers, many of whom left the company. A provision of the sales agreement – maintenance of health benefits – was arbitrarily discontinued for some. The new company folded within a year. Legal intervention became necessary.

Pat was furious. A company she'd nurtured for five years and which had become the standard of care for a large swath of Rhode Island's elderly was laid low in less than twelve months. A bitter pill to swallow.

Grandmother's Passing

In 1988 my mother, age 88, died of cardiac causes.

She had been an infrequent presence in my life. We never lived under the same roof until much later in her life. After a brief marriage to my father, she worked as a live-in housekeeper for a number of families on the East Side in Providence. That necessitated, very early on, that I move in with my father, his sister, and their mother in Pawtucket.

On Sunday afternoons during my grade and secondary school years, I took the bus into Providence and met my mother at the depot (now Kennedy Plaza). The routine seldom changed: a vanilla cabinet (milkshake) and chocolate éclair at a nearby Liggett's drugstore, then a movie. We often went to Fay's Theater, where after the movie, there was a vaudeville show. (Fay's Theater, I believe, was the last vaudeville house in the country.) The visit finished with a meal at Child's restaurant on Weybosset Street.

In summers, we moved from Pawtucket to Narragansett. My mother usually rented a cottage at Hurricane Village in Point Judith for a week, and I visited her there.

As mentioned earlier, my parents never divorced, and to my knowledge, my mother never had any boyfriends. More gregarious than my dad, she seemed better equipped to fill in with friends what certainly must have been some lonely times.

Much changed after I married and the kids came along. Pat was the main facilitator of the transition. Generous to a fault and unabashedly smitten with the children, my mother became a frequent visitor. Her arrival was always something of a happening, as though a small circus were coming to town. A few toots of the horn announced her arrival in a Studebaker loaded with toys. The kids appeared, and the party commenced.

In the process, my mother and I became better acquainted. There was no tearful do-over of the past or dramatic displays of affection, but rather a quiet reunion of two friends who had known each other for a long time and now, in trickles of small talk, were catching up on a life seldom shared.

Thanks to Pat and the kids, these were the best years of her life. I know – because she told me so.

A Century of Living

My aunt Bertha, my father's sister, was born in 1907 and died during her 101st year of natural causes. With her death went the toughest, mentally strongest woman I've ever known, and the most dominant influence in my life.

I came under my aunt's sway at a young age, probably around four, when I went to live with her, my grandmother, and my father.

Bertha, single and a public school teacher, acted as my surrogate mother; I was the son she never had. She was determined that the qualities she imagined for her son would be replicated in me – an impossible task, as she eventually found out, but that didn't prevent her from trying.

Education was her primary focus because she felt, with the right pieces of paper in hand, I could attain her definition of a successful life. That meant doing well in business and making a good wage. If she'd been asked who was the greater, more successful man, the Pope or John D. Rockefeller (choosing someone from her day), it would have been no contest. Although as a good Catholic she would not express it, I believe she felt that those who chose the religious life did so because they couldn't make it in the real world.

Very athletic, Bertha always involved me in whatever sport – swimming, skiing, badminton – she was participating in at the time. Even her choice of boyfriends had her nephew on the agenda. Matt Flynn, a classics professor at Providence College, tutored me in Latin; Frank Mason, an accountant, suffered through math; Mal Williams, a track coach at the University of Rhode Island, got me running; and Fritz Statler, who owned a biplane, took me aloft and introduced me to the basics of flying.

A remarkable woman in many ways, she deserves more than the few lines I can muster in this second book. But this can be said and it says it all: by the force of her personality and a determination which discouraged discussion, she insisted a young man unmoved by the sciences, with zero interest in medicine, become a physician. That would not have occurred without her. So over the years, whenever I had a bad day, there was always my aunt to blame.

BRANCHING OUT

Guard Duty

My affiliation with the National Guard had continued. Assigned to the 143rd Tactical Airlift Group at Quonset Point in North Kingstown, I worked in the hospital section, along with Dr. Blas Moreno. Blas, whom I became acquainted with during my residency at Memorial Hospital, was also a flight surgeon and commanded the medical unit.

Our flying time was accrued in the sturdy, dependable C-130 (Hercules) aircraft, the workhorse of the Air Force. Modified over the years, this four-engine turbo prop has served a variety of functions since its introduction in 1954: troop and cargo carrier, gunship, hurricane hunter, medivac, search and rescue, and aerial firefighting, to name a few. The plane remains in service, its short takeoff and landing capabilities especially suited for Middle East conflicts.

The Guard commitment included two weeks of active duty, which for our unit meant assignment to an Air Force hospital. There, working within our military medical classification, we were assimilated into the hospital structure.

An especially memorable stint was in June of 1980. We were assigned to Lajes AFB on the island of Terceira in the Azores. One of the nine islands in this Portuguese archipelago, Terceira had served as a mid-Atlantic gas station ever since planes had been flying between Europe and the States. (This role has markedly diminished with the advent of jet aircraft.)

The islands are of volcanic origin, and their position on either side of the Atlantic ridge – and the tectonic shifts in that region – make them especially vulnerable to earthquakes. In January of 1980, six months prior to our arrival, an earthquake (7.2 on the Richter scale) struck Terceira. There were 61 deaths, thousands injured, and a quarter of the buildings destroyed.

Within days of our arrival the island was hit again. Although moderate in intensity (3.1), the quake destroyed dozens of homes (many newly constructed) and hundreds were injured. There were no deaths.

The dispensary at the air base, and a nearby USN detachment, accommodated the overflow from the local civilian hospital. Our unit – thirty-five strong – supplanted their meager staff (two physicians, half-dozen nurses), and in effect, took over the operation of that facility. We remained in place until no longer needed. It was one of our more satisfying deployments.

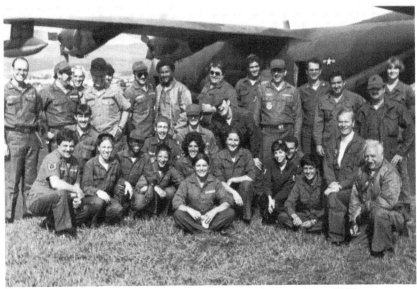

R.I. Air National Guard unit, departing Azores, June 1980

Shortly thereafter, Dr. Moreno was appointed the Rhode Island State Air Surgeon. Among other responsibilities, he served as medical advisor to the State Adjutant General. As a result of his ascendancy, I assumed his position as Commander of the 143rd TAC Hospital.

Sub Service

In the mid-1980s, while attending a drug company-sponsored cocktail party at the Larchwood Inn in Wakefield, I overheard a conversation: a medical director position was opening up at the Electric Boat (EB) Medical Dispensary, situated at Quonset Point in North Kingstown.

EB, a division of General Dynamics, operated out of two locations: Groton, Connecticut, and North Kingstown, Rhode Island. I knew little about the local facility, other than it built the hull sections for nuclear submarines, the final assembly accomplished at Groton. Tugs towing the barges on which the cylinders were secured were frequently seen on the bay.

Three days later, after much consideration, I decided to put my name into the mix of applicants. At that point in my medical career, I felt a change of pace was needed. To call it burnout seemed overly dramatic, but the practice – increasingly busy – was becoming a grind.

Writing about that time and aided by the clarity of hindsight, I think it was boredom more than stress or overwork. The practice had achieved an equilibrium, a predictable ebb and flow. With the occasional exception, medicine in the office setting tends to be a repetitive exercise. Perhaps that was the cause of my vague discontent. Whatever the reason, the thought of trying something new and different felt appealing.

I received an invitation to visit the dispensary, and to my surprise, I was greeted by Dr. Bart Sanders, whom I had worked with at URI health services and who had assumed my abbreviated North Kingstown practice. Bart was leaving the position there to begin an internal medicine residency at Roger Williams Hospital in Providence.

Bart outlined the duties of the position, the patient demographic, the relationship between management and the dispensary, and the experience of having a non-medical person as your supervisor. He offered a very positive assessment, emphasizing that his exit was for residency reasons and nothing beyond that. An interview was arranged with the human resources chief, Ron Smaldone.

Over lunch a few days later, Ron read through the job description and detailed the salary and benefits package. I had decided to work part time, at least to start, not wanting to put all my eggs in one basket in case the position didn't work out favorably. Mr. Smaldone didn't see that as a problem.

Later I was given a tour around the perimeter of the facility. Since I didn't have security clearance, I couldn't enter the buildings. Ron explained that EB had acquired the land – about 120 acres – after the Navy pulled out in 1973. Much of their work on the boats was done in former airplane hangars and warehouses. Paved slips, which the PBY amphibious aircraft used to come ashore, extended into the water. Barges were tied up at docks once occupied by the Atlantic Fleet during World War II.

"The hulls are built in sections," he explained, "three to a sub. Anything bigger, the barges couldn't handle. We package as much as we can, like piping, wiring, and hardware, into the hull sections before they're shipped to Groton. All the nuclear stuff goes in down there."

"Why don't they do it all there?" I asked.

"They're tight for space. They've run out of land. And the company's getting bigger."

When the tour ended, I expressed my thanks. As we said our good-byes, Ron mentioned I had to meet with the corporate medical director in Groton before any decision could be made. "But as far as I'm concerned, things look good," he added.

Pat drove down to Groton with me for the interview. Arriving early, we waited in the car outside the facility gates until the appointed time. Suddenly a blast came from a horn inside the facility. It was precisely noon. The gates opened, and a horde of workers streamed out, their destination a series of what appeared to be food trucks lined up along the street. What was being distributed, however, was not food but small bottles of booze.

"They have happy hour pretty early around here," Pat remarked.

I laughed. "Hey, like the song says, it's five o'clock somewhere."

She wished me luck, and I made my way through the workers to the gate and was escorted to the dispensary.

Dr. Kent was an older man who had been with the parent company, General Dynamics, for most of his medical life. He'd started his career in a family practice, and with that in common we had a pleasant, comfortable conversation.

The following week I was informed that the position was mine. My office schedule was reworked to allow twenty-five hours with EB.

quonsetgram

Quonset Ball Team New NE Champs

The Electric Boat/Quonset Point Industrial Softball Team has been basking in the warm glow of the champion's circle this week.

The team won the Northeastern Regional Major Men's Industrial Softball Tournament last weekend in Merrimac, New Hampshire.

The title came after five games. First, Quonset put away Boston Digital, 9-3, then First National Bank of Hartford, 4-0. Then it was a 2-1 win over Smith & Wesson and a 4-3 loss to the same team.

The title game, also against Smith & Wesson, was a rouser! Quonset, down 7-2 in the bottom of the final (seventh) inning, called up three pinch hitters. They started a rally and Quonset came out in front, 8-7.

"I still can't believe it," says Team Manager Bob Cambio. "The whole team was outstanding! In the final minutes of that last game we got eight straight hits!"

The win qualifies the team to travel to Atlanta, Georgia over Labor Day Weekend to compete in national competition.

Vans Are Open

Why not commute in comfort? And at less cost, too! The QuonseTrans van program has these openings:

Providence on the third shift and two vans from Newport on the second shift.

If you're interested, call the QuonseTrans office on 2296.

The program now has 29 vans operating from three states.

New Medical Director Named

Quonset has a new medical director. He's Dr. Eugene B. McKee of Narragansett.

Dr. McKee comes to the facility from a family practice in Wakefield.

A Pawtucket native, he is a graduate of Holy Cross College and the Royal College of Physicians and Surgeons (Dublin, Ireland and London, England) and interned at Pawtucket's Memorial Hospital.

McKee, who also served as an Air Force flight surgeon from 1963-1966, says he's "looking forward to practicing preventive medicine here," especially in the fields of cardio-vascular problems, emphysema, diabetes and glaucoma.

He and his wife, Patricia, have five children.

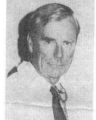

Dr. Eugene McKee

Don't Gamble With Radiation

ground; magenta symbol and letters) around the facility, remember that it means precisely what it says: "Keep Out."

There's a good reason for that. The sign's used to indicate areas where industrial radiography (radiation inspection) is going on.

The sign's usually attached to a magenta-striped bright yellow rope or cloth tape barrier that cordons off an entire area. Look for flashing red lights at gates, too. All these things signal you to stay away from the area.

The areas are marked by the industrial radiography which identifies, segregates and controls (See GAMBLE, Page 2)

If you come across the sign above (bright yellow back-

The dispensary was nicely appointed and well-staffed with a receptionist/secretary, X-ray capability, on-site audiologist, and blood draw station; physiotherapy was contracted with an outside group. Two full-time nurses covered the day shift and one the second shift.

Physical examinations, either OSHA – mandated or a requirement of a particular occupation (e.g., radiation workers and commercial drivers), were done on a periodic basis. Pre-employment physicals that included a drug screen were accomplished as necessitated by hiring demands. Shortly after my arrival, I instituted an executive physical program which included cardiac stress testing.

The acute injuries presenting in the dispensary were, due to the nature of the work, mainly of the musculoskeletal variety, with low back complaints heading the list. Those of a more chronic nature usually had an ergonomic etiology. Welders and grinders frequently presented with eye injuries: most commonly, imbedded corneal foreign bodies and flash burns which occurred when eyes were inadvertently exposed to the UV light of a welding torch. Dr. Sanders had arranged for the purchase of a slit lamp, which allowed the majority of cases to be handled in-house. Those requiring further treatment were referred to Drs. Coghlin and Asher, ophthalmologists in Wickford.

When the facility chief, Bill Bennett, and I had our introductory conversation, he expressed quite forcibly his wish for increased emphasis on worker health issues and accident prevention programs in the facility. He rattled off a list of statistics detailing lost work days because of injuries, specifically noting those which extended beyond two weeks, which he categorized as chronic. He stated his support for any initiatives which would impact these unacceptable stats.

Over the ensuing months, various interventions were put in place: smoking cessation programs offered twice a year; favorable membership fees at various health clubs in the state; articles addressing health issues placed in the "Quonsetgram," the weekly facility newsletter; departmental "Waist Away" weight-loss competitions; dietary counseling; and 5K road races. Safety, health, and substance abuse talks were given to both employees and management on a regular basis.

Part of my job was gaining the trust of the worker and not coming across as the "company doc" who automatically took the side of management when it came to work-related issues. When an employee reported a job-associated injury or complaint to his supervisor, the tendency was to fault the employee. The standard response was that if the worker "had been more careful" or "paid more attention," the incident wouldn't have happened.

It was a tough sell convincing management that in the majority of cases, the cause lay not with the employee but with the demands of the assigned job and/or the environment in which they were asked to work. Any injury that didn't relate to a specific event (e.g., foreign body in an eye or a sprained ankle), was viewed with suspicion. The concept of cumulative trauma – which accounted for most of the long-term disability cases – was met with skepticism. Yet jobs that involved eight hours of repetitive hand motion (painter. secretary, or grinder), or occupations that required constant lifting or working in an enclosed space during the heat of summer, were examples of scenarios that increased the out-of-work statistic.

The inference that most workers were looking to acquire an injury severe enough to put them out of work and thus be eligible for Workers Compensation payments, was not a productive approach. Albeit not totally out of line. Many workers found their "Dr. Summeroff," a title attached to those physicians liberally dispensing out-of-work notes for extended periods, often for minor injuries. But that was a relatively small worker bloc.

The concept that a flawed process, not the worker, was the primary cause of accidents in the workplace, had been articulated most prominently by Edward Deming and Joseph Duran, American industrial engineers/statisticians shortly after World War II. Their premise was that rarely could injuries be attributed to a lack of skill or motivation in the worker. Whether welders, physicians, airline pilots, or high-wire workers, people generally went to work each day with the idea of doing a good job. Their intent was not to fail – or fall. It was found that when workers were demonstrably to blame, it was often the case of poor job design, failure of leadership, or unclear communication relative to job objectives.

> **An aside:** *Deming felt that 85% of car defects were due to the mistakes of management, engineers, designers, and those who supplied the auto parts. Their theories of total quality improvement (TQI), though rejected by American industry, were embraced (with extraordinary results) by the Japanese. It was felt that the principles they formulated provided the philosophy and model for the unprecedented level of quality and productivity of today's Japanese industries. No longer were their products synonymous with junk. A decade passed before American cars began to catch up, finally overcoming the impact of a sclerotic upper management and union intransigence.*

Deming and Duran's approach: once the problem has been identified, all aspects of the work process are identified. This involves discussion crossing multiple lines of authority, from production worker to upper management. Most importantly: involve the workers, educate them as to company goals (e.g., zero defects), and empower them. If an employee recognizes a problem on the assembly line, allow him to shut it down (and they often did) until the concern is resolved. Quality circles are developed: groups of workers meeting with management, suggesting ways to improve the product.

This was the tactic we adopted related to injuries at Electric Boat – specifically, for those disabilities which removed people from the workplace for a significant period of time. The dispensary, working in conjunction with the safety department, conducted workplace evaluations until we came up with the probable reason for the incident. The investigation was done in the company of the worker, whose typical comment at the end of our review was, "I could have told you guys what the problem was. I tried to tell the boss." Conversations continued with the employee regarding their suggestions for improvement, preferably with their supervisor not present, to remove the intimidation factor.

A series of meetings were arranged by Mr. Bennett with all supervisors in attendance. Results, without pointing fingers, were discussed, along with ways to improve the work process in their departments. Many bosses didn't buy it and took a defensive position, still blaming the worker. Mr. Bennett insisted that the recommendations be implemented. All complied.

Changes included a number of ergonomic interventions; rotating work assignments (a four-hour time limit in repetitive work situations); increased use of machines in frequent or heavy lifting situations; two work breaks, ten minutes each, during an eight-hour shift; and dispensary notification of any joint complaint, no matter how minor. We included the suggestions of unnamed workers. A follow-up meeting in thirty days was scheduled for each department.

As a result, two outcomes were noted: improved communication between the workforce and the Medical and Safety departments, and a decrease in the number of lost-time injuries. Bill Bennett was pleased.

A Hospital Is Not a Factory (Nor Patients Toyotas)

In the fall of 1987 I received an invitation to lunch from Donald Mazzarelli, the CEO of South County Hospital. We met at what is currently the Mariner Grille. Halfway through our Bloody Marys, Don asked if I would be interested in heading up the Quality Assurance (QA) program at the hospital. My answer was an emphatic "no."

Dismissing my reply, he mentioned that I could basically make my own schedule. "Of course, there are mandatory meetings, usually early morning, which shouldn't affect your office hours." Mr. Mazzarelli outlined his expectations for the position and promised clerical help. The last sip of the Bloody Mary coincided with my agreement to try the position for three months.

My responsibilities as director were to maintain patient care standards, coordinate the monitoring and evaluation activities of the various clinical departments, and identify opportunities to improve patient care. Peer review and physician credentialing also fell under my purview. The position served as liaison between the medical staff, hospital administration, and the board of trustees. The most significant responsibility was to ensure that the hospital was in compliance with the standards of medical care as outlined by the Joint Commission of Hospital Accreditation (JCAHO). Inspectors from that organization descend on hospitals at regular intervals to bestow (or not) their imprimatur of approval.

To the extent possible, I tried to incorporate the TQI model used at Electric Boat into the hospital setting. Imperfect processes relative to delivery of health services can be readily identified: missing lab or X-ray reports, medical record dictation glitches, poor communication between nursing shifts, cold and unpalatable food, physician on-call systems gone awry, and the myriad of other areas which detract from a hospital's quality and efficiency.

The difficulty in applying the industrial model to service organizations is the intrusion of the human element. A hospital is not a factory, and patients are not Toyotas. The treatment process in any given hospital death may be totally correct, and yet the "product" has an untoward outcome. Aside from these exceptions, the hospital proved an ideal workplace to implement the TQI model.

The job appealed to me. Although reviewing records can be a tedious chore, I enjoyed my involvement with the departments, working with them to identify areas of their clinical or administrative services which either didn't meet JCAHO standards or the department identified as needing a fix. Indicators of optimal performance were agreed upon, and each assigned a threshold which had to be met or exceeded before the problem area could be considered resolved. Department records were monitored for three months, the results tabulated and presented to the department for further action as required.

While I had, with the assistance of a knowledgeable and efficient secretary (Mary Hayes), eased into my new role with a minimum of transition difficulties, Donald Mazzarelli's tenure as CEO had become contentious, a road riven with obstacles. His situation was doubtless made more difficult by having to follow in the long shadow of Donald Ford.

Heroes, it is said, know when to die, and perhaps successful CEOs know when to leave. No amount of legerdemain would have excluded South County Hospital from the economic forces buffeting every other hospital in the state and nation during that period. The budget surplus for the hospital in 1987 became a $500,000 deficit in 1988, due in large measure to shortfalls in Medicare reimbursement. Statewide hospitals were expected to lose $20 million over the same period. Mr. Mazzarelli's management style and methods may have grated, but his goals were realistic and his options to accomplish them limited.

Other factors added to the mix of discontent: two upper-management employees were fired as a cost-saving measure; an early retirement plan was offered, which thirty-five employees (including health providers) accepted; nurses petitioned for union representation; and physicians voiced accreditation concerns – all ingredients for a simmering rebellion. Meetings were held with everyone concerned and alternatives explored. Compromises were made, but at the end of the day, Don was asked to resign by the board of trustees. In August of 1989, he did.

In an effort to calm the roiling waters, the trustees, in an astute move, chose Ralph Misto to replace Mr. Mazzarelli. Ralph was a known entity and familiar with hospital operations. Originally brought on board by Don Ford as chief of laboratories in 1966, he served as director of personnel and eventually vice president for management services in the mid-1970s.

Changes required to address the difficulties of any organization are more palatable when presented in a transparent and forthright manner by someone whom the employees know has their best interests and those of the institution at heart. This was what Ralph brought to the table. Credibility was restored, morale improved, and in time, so too, did the bottom line. The Donald (Ford) couldn't have done it better.

During my last year (1992) as quality assurance director, the hospital was notified that we could expect a JCAHO accreditation visit during the late summer or fall. Mary Swanson, RN, was assigned to the QA department in preparation for the visit.

During our initial conversation, we defined our roles: Mary would involve herself with nursing functions, while I would handle physician accreditation and the clinical departments. Mary and I worked well together. Her efforts were invaluable.

In October 1992, the examiners spent the better part of a week with us. The visit went well. The hospital was awarded Accreditation with Commendation which, according to JCAHO, "is the highest accreditation decision awarded to a hospital that has demonstrated exemplary performance." This was the first such designation for South County Hospital and an honor conferred on less than 5 percent of hospitals in the country.

My three-month work trial with QA had extended to six years. A Peter Allen song lyric, popular at the time, decreed, "It's best to leave when you're in love." Paraphrased to "when you're on top," it seemed to make sense in my situation. After a farewell drink with Mary Swanson, during which, with humor and exaggeration, we replayed our successful efforts, I bid adieu to the great experience that was the quality assurance program at SCH.

Urgent Care Calls

Some months later, Dr. John Brady, the medical director at South County Hospital's Treatment Center in North Kingstown, offered me a part-time position working with him. Urgent care was a branch of medicine I hadn't been involved in previously, which was an attraction. I accepted and with some juggling of the schedule, continued my hours with Electric Boat and a scaled-down office practice.

A highly efficient staff (the nurses all graduates of excellent training programs), made the transition pleasant and seamless. Some aspects of urgent care that surprised me: the large volume, the diversity of pathology, and the acuity of many presenting complaints. Patients presented with symptoms (chest pain and shortness of breath, for example) that I assumed would have brought them to a hospital emergency room. When asked why they passed by the Miriam and Rhode Island Hospitals on the way to our facility, the usual reply was that they didn't want to be sitting for hours in a waiting room, wished to be closer to home and liked the nurses at the Treatment Center. (I'm sure they meant to say doctors.)

Dr. Brady was one of the best clinicians I've worked with over the years. And he wasn't the type to crow loudly when he aced you on a diagnosis. One example: a healthy-appearing twenty-year-old male presented with a throbbing, intensely itchy foot.

He offered this history: "Been in Barbados the last couple of weeks. Barefoot kind of holiday. Did a lot of scuba stuff. Think I scratched it on some coral. The pain is getting so bad I can't sleep."

On his right sole were four raised, red, angry-looking welts with what looked like reddish brown threads extending into the surrounding tissue. The entire undersurface of the foot was puffy.

"Putting alcohol on them makes them worse," the young man added.

Though not the typical presentation, I assumed the cause was related to the coral scratch history, breaks in the skin that had allowed infection to develop. I wrote a prescription. "Not any better in twenty-four hours," I advised, "come back."

The desk John and I shared had the usual clutter when I returned to work two days later and sat down to review the previous day's lab and X-ray reports. To clear some room, I pushed aside an open dermatology book. Displayed on the page was a picture of a rash almost identical to the one I had seen two days earlier. The caption beneath read, "Cutaneous larva migrans."

The penny dropped, the light went on. Without fanfare, a subtle "gotcha" from the good Dr. B.

The young man, I learned, had indeed returned in twenty-four hours, and Dr. Brady corrected my impression. The clue to the diagnosis was the history of walking barefoot in a subtropical area, where hookworm larvae residing in the sand or soil can burrow into the skin and inflame the tissue. Over the next three years I saw two patients presenting with similar scenarios; they thought me quite clever when I rendered my opinion. John wasn't around then, but I thanked him anyway.

After we had worked together for approximately three years, Dr. Brady became ill. Following treatment and a period of time out of work, he returned to the Treatment Center; shortly thereafter, John left the practice of medicine. It marked the loss of an outstanding physician and good friend.

I moved into Dr. Brady's full-time position as medical director which meant, after twenty-one years, parting ways with Electric Boat and a quarter century of private practice.

Formerly a Lum's restaurant, the Treatment Center didn't begin its days as a medical facility with an ideal structural footprint. Patient flow wasn't optimal. The waiting room was inadequate and misplaced, but I thought its location neutralized the architectural shortcomings. Located on busy Post Road in North Kingstown, near the entrance to the expanding Quonset Point industrial park, it provided a well-equipped facility equally responsive to both the industrial and community population. Dr. Bart Sanders, now a board-certified internist, joined our staff a short time later.

Dr. Brady's goal had been to present to the public a "one-stop shopping" experience, to the extent that the patient, upon leaving the building, had received a diagnosis, appropriate treatment, and a follow-up plan. If further interventions were needed (e.g., radiological, laboratory, or a specialist consultation), that process would have also been set in motion. Orthopedic and radiological input relative to questionable bone and joint injuries was to be obtained before the patient exited the facility. This comprehensive approach was continued during my years at the Treatment Center.

On the occupational side, multiple companies utilized us for their pre-employment physicals or as required by state or federal mandate. In most instances each of these categories required a drug screen.

In order to avoid legal questions down the road, all involved in the drug testing process, from the person who collected the urine to the doctor who interpreted the results, had to obtain certification as to their ability to perform their particular task. For the physician, that required attendance at a two-day educational program, at the end of which an exam was given. On successful completion, you were certified as a Medical Review Officer (MRO).

The seminar devoted considerable time to evaluation of the employee who presented during work with bizarre or unusual behavior. Cases were cited in which drugs or alcohol were assumed to be the cause. The individuals, often young, showed obvious signs of impairment – couldn't walk a straight line, unable to recite the alphabet or count backwards – and occasionally were violent. In most instances the employee was sent home, sometimes fired, and frequently the police became involved. The problems, as the study went on to illustrate, were not due to drugs or alcohol, but a medical condition gone awry, and in one instance, sequelae of head trauma. Rather than home or the police station, the individual should have been sent to the hospital. Death occurred in one instance, litigation in all.

The moral of the story: the employer (and police) need to be careful not to automatically ascribe unusual behavior to drugs or alcohol, even if its odor is obvious.

One of the companies in the industrial park, Job Lot, attuned to this possibility and the legal implications, asked that a discussion on the topic be arranged for their supervisors. On a half dozen occasions, I gave presentations to management outlining the proper approach to an employee who was acting strangely. Among the most important questions to be asked of the individual: "Are you taking any medication?" and "Are you a diabetic?" As an MRO, I was permitted to issue certificates to those who attended the training. The pro-active stance of the organization, its foresight and awareness, was commendable.

Doctor at Sea

Sometime during late 1997, I came across a magazine article which discussed the role of the ship doctor in the cruise industry. The writer briefly outlined physician responsibilities, and in more expansive fashion, the delights of ocean travel. The article finished with a mailing address for physicians considering such a position. It sounded intriguing. I sent them my CV and thought little more about it.

Three years later, I received a call asking if I would be interested in working a five-day Caribbean cruise sailing out of New Orleans. There were two cruise dates available. The first offering didn't allow enough time to work out practice coverage. The second was doable, so I signed on as ship's physician on the

Commodore Cruise Line's *Enchanted Capri*, scheduled to sail to the Caribbean on October 7.

The cruise line arranged a flight from Providence and a hotel in one of the city's less attractive areas. Midafternoon the following day, I boarded the ship and found my way to the dispensary. The nurse welcomed me. In the course of our chat, I learned she was from Tennessee and had worked for eight years as the ship's nurse. Her husband worked in the ship's kitchen. Tall and gangly, she wore her hair parted in the middle and tied into a bun. Her strong Southern accent had a Jim Nabors sing-song quality.

As we were chatting, the phone rang. The conversation was brief. A man apparently had fallen off a stool at the deck bar and was unable to stand up. We both responded, she with her emergency bag.

The man was heavyset and swarthy, his shirt soaked in sweat as he lay on his back, conscious but not moving.

"Any chest pain?" I asked.

He shook his head no.

"Trouble breathing? Any heart problems?"

He answered no to both. "Just blood pressure," he replied.

His lungs were clear. Heart rate was quick. Blood pressure low. He looked scared. In spite of his full color, there was a grayness around his lips and eyes.

"Do you have an EKG?" I asked the nurse. She nodded yes and hurried off to the dispensary, returning with it in a matter of minutes.

Although only a three-lead tracing with much artifact, two of the three leads had obvious ischemic changes. That was enough for me. "We've got to get this guy to a hospital."

"We can't," she answered. "We've left the dock."

Indeed, we were slipping quietly down the Mississippi toward the Gulf.

"This happens a lot," she assured me. "Drinking in the sun, all the heat. We'll take him downstairs and get an IV going."

I looked at the man. Sweat was still dripping off his chin. He was starting to become agitated but made no move to stand up. Still no pain.

"Okay, we'll do the IV. But this guy's got to get off the ship. Tell the captain that. I will if you don't want to." I thought to myself, *I'm sure'n hell not going to spend the next five days with this guy on board.*

She called the bridge. I could hear the eruption at the other end of the line. About five minutes later, the ship started to slow and then turn – a tricky operation, given the narrowness of the river and the traffic. The ship's horn blared through the entire maneuver.

The nurse placed an IV while I spoke to the man's wife. She was distraught but agreed totally with the decision to get him off the ship. She was very grateful. "He doesn't drink, by the way," she added.

We were met at the dock by an ambulance, and he was whisked away to Charity Hospital.

The nurse remained very upset with me for the remainder of the cruise. When I did meet the captain, however, he made no mention of the incident. Nor did I learn how the man made out. But there I was, my bags not yet unpacked, turning liners around on the Mississippi. It was my Walter Mitty moment.

The Mississippi cruise was my first and last as a ship's doctor. There was no further communication with the Commodore Line. I think the nurse in some fashion nixed any return possibilities. Part of the reason, I believe, was that the dispensary was her baby, and she didn't want interlopers invading her space. For her, the physician was an unfortunate requirement which satisfied maritime law.

The take-home message for physicians interested in working the cruise lines, at least based on my brief experience: there is no *Love Boat* scenario. The physician is always on call, with responsibility for both passengers and crew. The social amenities of the cruise are scarcely enjoyed.

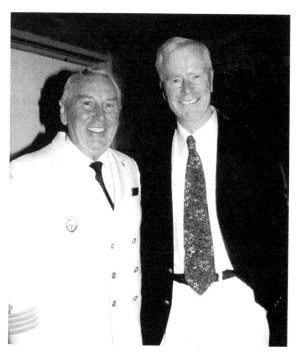

Captain of the *Enchanted Capri*
and the author in 2000

Calling It Quits

Word of the urgent care facility's relocation to East Green-wich came down from hospital administration in 2007. It seemed a good time to notify Lou Giancola, Hospital President and CEO, that I would be stepping down as medical director and assuming a lighter schedule as soon as a replacement was found.

We moved into the new facility in 2008. Whereas the Treatment Center lacked the ideal floor plan, our new digs – bright, roomy, and nicely appointed – were designed with our specific function and needs in mind.

In short order, it became apparent that the move was a wise one. A new patient demographic was introduced to our services, with a corresponding increase in urgent care volume and utilization of our travel clinic and outpatient services.

Dr. Sandra Johnson came aboard as director in 2010 and remained with us for approximately a year before deciding to pursue another career opportunity. Dr. Joseph Turner, an internist, succeeded her as medical director. In the course of our conversations, we agreed on a significant decrease in my hours. Thus began my inexorable retreat from the practice of medicine, which – with a smidgen of relief – ended in January of 2013 with my retirement.

Funny How Things Happen Sometimes

As I considered what might ease the boredom of retirement years, I knew that clinical medicine, in any capacity, would not be among the choices. One option: during my years in private practice I had been certified to perform Class 1 FAA (commercial pilot) flight physicals. As one of the few with this qualification in southern Rhode Island, I had acquired a sizable clientele.

With the thought of maintaining that peripheral connection to medicine, I made plans to attend an FAA refresher seminar in Boston, after which I would apply to have my certification reinstated.

The seminar was informative; there had been many regulatory and procedural changes since my departure. At the close of the weekend assembly, a small ceremony was held to recognize physician-examiners who had performed with the agency for a considerable length of time. I paid little attention until I noticed one recipient departing the stage with his award. There was something familiar about him. A beard obscured his face; he walked with a slight limp. I watched as he returned to his seat in the front row. A woman turned toward him and kissed his cheek. Her face came into view, as did a wedge of white in her dark, gray hair. *I'll be damned, the woman back in Texas. The dance hall.*

Laura, Rob, and I had a brief reunion a few minutes later. Three months after leaving Texas he had gone back to the old red barn looking for her. ("I told you there was something special about that place.") She didn't work there any longer, but he tracked her down. A courtship followed, they married and had four children. Their home was in Honolulu and they were heading back that night. We promised to stay in touch.

I have always been struck by how the most benign of decisions can have such lasting implications. In this instance, Rob's suggestion that night of a left turn rather than a right, changed the course of his life. Perhaps it's all pre-determined, part of God's Grand Design, as the Jesuits would argue back in my Holy Cross days. But it is funny how things happen sometimes.

Patients Remembered

As I chatted with one of the nurses during my final week, she asked, "After all these years in practice, there must be some things that stand out, patients you'll never forget, catastrophes you've escaped" – she paused – "or didn't."

"As far as disasters," I answered, "thanks to a worn out guardian angel, I've been lucky. As far as the other stuff, things pretty much blend over the years. Nothing really stands out. Medicine, at least in the office, is a pretty humdrum deal."

I knew this wasn't totally true, but I hadn't thought enough about the question to give a good answer.

I suppose I could have mentioned the lady who had her baby in one of the exam rooms, or the pregnant woman back in my residency days who, after a middle-of-the-night delivery, wouldn't stop bleeding (due to a clotting defect, we later learned). The exertions required of the nurse and me...how lucky we were to stop the flow...are fixed in memory.

Then there was the patient with an inflatable penile prosthesis that had been placed three months earlier. The deflation valve had stuck, and the fluid in the cylinder couldn't drain off. When I saw him in the waiting room on a warm August afternoon with a coat draped over his lap, I knew something was up.

But after my retirement, as thoughts of writing about the early times took shape, three patients came to mind. Their stories were neither a feather in my cap – a daunting diagnosis, a life-saving intervention – nor a clinical embarrassment, but rather patients whose stories had a quality, be it humor, pathos, or eccentricity, which made them memorable.

The Call of the Sea

My friend Pete (name altered) and I worked together at the Point Judith Fisherman Co-operative during our late teens, filleting fish (primarily flounder and sole). Mine was a summer job, but Pete had worked there year-round since his graduation from high school. During my last summer at the co-op, he left and began working on the fishing boats.

Mention should be made of the unfortunate downside of cutting fish, at least for a young man interested in the opposite sex.

The smell acquired, impervious to deodorants, showers, and an impressive array of soaps, curtailed nearly all relationships with women (and presumably men). My own family, unless it were raining, insisted I change my clothes and take my meals outside the house. The three summers I was involved in that occupation were a void – perhaps "more of a void" would be the more precise terminology – in my dating life, a psychological consequence that took years to overcome. There were two exceptions: you could date a female cutter (there was one, and I did) with the expectation that the odors would neutralize each other. To some extent that was true, but the amount of perfume she used as an adjunctive measure made it hard to catch my breath – at least, I think that was the reason. The other possibility: find someone with a chronic sinus condition.

Crewmen on the boats back in the late 1950s, even those new to the job, such as Pete, took home some serious money – in the precincts of $2,000 for a two-week trip. Unfortunately for many, the cash never made it that far. Once ashore, the next port of call for many was the Bon Vue Inn, a local watering hole.

Tall, blonde, lean, and usually with a fine-looking woman in tow, Pete was an active player in drinking stints starting at the Vue and often extending to Jamestown and Newport. Sessions, depending on the amount of cash and stamina available, stretched for days. He visited me a time or two at the co-op, recounting his latest adventure, of which he usually had little memory. Going on the boats, he said, was the best move he'd ever made. He had found his niche: the camaraderie, the hard work, of course the money, and tellingly, the long stretches at sea had turned his life around. The booze, the drugs, even the women, he said, were just distractions, a bit of the blaze and brawl, until he got back to the sea.

After being away from the area for a number of years, I lost contact with Pete but heard that he had married and settled down. A couple of years into my practice, he dropped by to see me. He still had the looks, with a few more sun creases around the eyes and the hollows of his cheeks a little deeper, but his broad, angled features remained taut and furrow-free. He confirmed his marriage and told of his two beautiful daughters. Now, with his own boat and the fish running well, life was good. He was taking courses at the Maritime Academy at Buzzards Bay on Cape Cod. "I want to be a master mariner someday, work the big boats. Only thing, Doc," he said, getting to the reason for his visit, "I get nervous when I'm home. Drive the wife crazy. Mean to the kids I love to death. Maybe you can give me something to calm me down a little." Which I did.

A few weeks later, his wife "Sally" met with me at the office. Pete had asked her to come by, she said, so I could hear her side of the story and possibly offer advice as to what they should do next. Recalling the women Pete had squired around back in the day, her appearance surprised me. Of medium height, with a full figure and a face free of makeup, she wore a plain, loose-fitting dress, her gray hair, carelessly combed, was gathered in a bun.

Sally confirmed what Pete had told me of his behavior. "It sometimes gets pretty bad," she said. "The kids get frightened. I tell them Daddy works hard, and sometimes he brings his weariness home. I ask them to be patient with him."

"What seems to set him off?" I asked.

"Nothing I know of. It starts like clockwork, three to four days after a trip. He gets antsy and begins drinking."

Rather than an angry, vindictive wife whose life and that of her kids was being disrupted by her husband's behavior, Sally seemed more a concerned mother speaking of an unruly child acting out, going through a phase that would pass.

"How's he on the boat?" I asked. "Have you heard?"

"Fine, no drinking. His crew tells me he's the most easygoing captain they've ever worked for."

"It's the damndest thing," Pete said when I saw him again. "As soon as I clear the breakwater it drains out of me, this tension. Out of sight of land, I'm a new person. I call home and apologize for the misery I caused. But Sally's great, tells me everything's fine, and she's glad I'm feeling better."

Pete's DNA, it seemed, got stuck at some evolutionary synapse before we morphed into terrestrials. This is not unique, I've since learned, especially among the cruising community. From solo sailors to families, they follow a loose, weather-dependent itinerary, occasionally hooking up with their vagabond brethren at a favored port. After a few days with their fellow sailors and a brief dalliance with Mother Earth, they escape with the tide and head back to sea.

Pilots often recollect similar feelings when they have "slipped the surly bonds of earth." The French writer and aviator Saint-Exupery spent his life writing about that very topic.

The medication I prescribed for Pete took the edge off his anxiety and helped him sleep but was only a Band Aid. I had suggested counselling during both their visits, but Pete dismissed this with a flip comment along the lines of, "Real men don't do that stuff."

Then he changed his mind. A consultation was set up. Sally, however, wasn't in agreement, feeling they could work things out themselves. Perhaps Sally was happy with the situation, and somehow she liked the way things were. This can be seen in those who care for ill spouses, alcoholics, substance abusers, or individuals, who for whatever reason, aren't making it on their own. The caregivers play a key role in the lives of those so afflicted. If the illness or abuse problem resolves, their importance, power, and control are gone. They are no longer needed; no longer a somebody. I suspected some variation of that dynamic was going on with Sally. Pete went to the appointment by himself.

Unfortunately, Pete's home situation didn't improve. One of the children appeared at school with a bruise. She told the teacher she was "rough-housing with Daddy." An investigation ensued, and a restraining order was issued. Sally did not press charges, but the publicity continued. She decided to leave the area and divorced Pete. Custody arrangements for the children were worked out. Pete was heartbroken.

The turn of fortune took its toll on Pete: brilliant blue eyes were lost in puffy pouches, his face was bearded and bloated, teeth in need of repair. He worked when he was able. The biggest hurt: only seeing his daughters twice a month, each visit restricted to three hours after driving two hundred miles. Even then, he wasn't sure they wanted him there – and was afraid to ask.

Things improved when he got his master mariner's license. Jobs took him to all corners of the globe. As a member of the upper strata, the elite of the shipping industry, he began to act and look the part. Never one to drink aboard ship, his three-months-on and one-month-off rotation slimmed him down and sobered him up. His face reappeared, and his brain dried out. More importantly, he reconciled with his daughters, now in their twenties. He knew they were sincere because they asked to visit him in Rhode Island. Sally had remarried an old school chum.

During his vacation month, Pete always came back to Galilee and Point Judith. Sometimes he hooked up with a boat, working as a crew member just to get off land for a while. One squally fall day somewhere off the Grand Banks, the boat he was working on was violently swept up in a storm. Quite rapidly – within thirty minutes – the boat went keel up and sank. The two survivors of the crew of six said they last saw Pete swimming toward a crew member struggling in the waves.

His name was etched, along with other fishermen lost at sea, on one of the stone tablets at the Fishermen's Memorial near Point Judith. Seeing it, I was struck by the irony: the same ocean that had brought him to life and sustained him had, just as capriciously, taken it away. Probably, if he were given the choice, he would have had it no other way.

"Sea Fever," John Masefield's reflection on those hardy souls who spend their lives on the ocean, is also inscribed on a tablet at the site. The poem's lines *"... the call of the running tide, a wild call, a clear call that may not be denied,"* seemed a perfect epitaph for my old friend Pete.

The Doctor and the Businessman

During the mid-1990s, Dr. Jack Turco, a general practitioner, became a patient. A physician with an outsized personality, he had retired from active practice some ten years earlier. Although Jack would be considered one of the "Old Guard" in the chronological sense – probably in his early fifties when I came to town in 1970—he was an infrequent presence in the hospital and not involved in any of the political machinations of the entrenched group.

While in medical school at Georgetown University and during his post-graduate training, he paid some of his tuition by playing professional football for the Washington Redskins under an assumed name. Medical training finished, he returned to Rhode Island and opened a general practice in his home on High Street in Peace Dale, Rhode Island.

My first contact with Jack was during my early teenage years when, on many occasions, I caddied for him at the Point Judith Country Club. He was an excellent golfer – handicap in the single digits for most of his playing days – with a full, fluid swing that was compared to that of Sammy Snead. Occasionally his round was interrupted by a caddy running out from the clubhouse to tell him he was needed at the hospital. If this interruption happened when he was losing his match, opponents were convinced his exit was somehow prearranged.

Significant exchanges of money were common in the four-somes Jack played with on weekends. A fifty-dollar Nassau – the amount bet on the match play outcome for the front nine, back nine, and total eighteen holes – was not uncommon. With side bets (presses) along the way, the winnings or losings could easily extend into several hundreds of dollars for each player, which at that time was a significant amount of money. A very competitive Jack Turco, it was said, made more hitting a golf ball on weekends than he did from five days of pushing pills.

An aside: Ben Tallman was the golf professional at Point Judith during my caddying days. For two summers I was his chosen caddy (something of an honor in those days), shagging balls in the morning when he gave lessons and carrying his bag for afternoon matches.

A substantial portion of Ben's income was derived from wagers made on the course. Weekends were his show time, when the heavy rollers came to town. Significant amounts of cash – into the thousands, some said – passed hands over the course of those two days. Dev Milburn, a nationally ranked polo player and an excellent golfer, was a regular in these foursomes. (Jack Turco was well able to compete with this group, but the freight was a bit too heavy if he had a bad day.)

Ben was a canny golfer. Not long off the tee – but always on the fairway – he made amends with his short game. Within 150 yards of the green, he was a master. Besides knowing the golf course, he was imperturbable. Dev occasionally won, but over the course of a summer he paid a heavy price for his weekend jousts with the pro. (It was said – and I believe it to be true – that Ben arranged with the greens keeper, "Old Man" Coulter, favorable cup placement in preparation for his match later in the day).

Ben insisted that bets be settled at the end of play. Although invited, he never joined the members for post-match drinks. The member/employee line was never crossed. So just off the eighteenth green, under the shade of a tree, some large bills changed hands. Ben carried a wad of cash, bound by an elastic band, in his pocket, and although I never saw the transactions, I knew who won and who lost the matches. Very few bills were ever peeled off Ben's stash.

The Point Judith Country Club, founded in 1894 by Philip Syng Physick (his golfing attire: usually a natty combination of construction boots and overalls), was at that time, a very Waspish enclave for the affluent golfer. Jack was the first Italian-American member, his admission facilitated by a patient who played there. Over the years much of his practice derived from his membership at Point Judith and the equally exclusive Dunes Club. His was a concierge practice long before the term was used to describe a health coverage option. Although an excellent revenue source, the carriage trade can be demanding, as I found out during the times I covered his practice. If Mrs. X's B-12 shot was scheduled for noon, a 12:15 arrival was not acceptable. A midnight bout of vomiting required immediate attention. Getting caught up in the lifestyles of the rich and famous could be a draining distraction.

When Dr. Turco phased out his practice in the early 1980s, he referred most of his remaining patients to me. One was Carl (name and details altered), a successful, seventy-five-year-old businessman who lived out on Moonstone Beach. According to Jack's notes, he was in excellent physical condition, active mentally and physically, and abstinent of alcohol and tobacco. His visits to me were for relatively minor complaints. A tidy, small man with wary blue eyes behind black-rimmed glasses, Carl always gave the impression that my medical opinion was being taken under advisement. As my secretary noted, Carl was not used to sitting in a waiting room for extended periods; the frequent trips to the magazine rack, she noted, betrayed his impatience. But over the course of a couple of years, we got along well.

From the lifestyle he pursued to the car he drove, Carl's wealth was never marked by ostentation or a preening superiority. Any flaunting was low key: a quietly arranged flight to Bermuda on the company jet with a few friends to play a round of golf, with a return home by evening, was more his style.

One afternoon at the end of an office visit with Carl, the conversation turned to Dr. Turco, who had recently been hospitalized. Carl was concerned, as for many years Jack had been a good friend and understanding physician. About to leave, Carl asked me if Jack had ever mentioned their first meeting. I shook my head.

"Sort of interesting," he said. Leaning back in the exam room chair, a bemused smile on his face, he began: "I was about forty-five years old, working hard, trying to get my business going, wife, three kids, the usual home stuff. I had just come off a couple of bad business deals. A lot of anxiety. But I was used to that. Then came the depression. Ever been depressed, Doc?"

"Sure, at times," I said, "but nothing too serious."

Carl leaned forward, elbows on his knees, hands clasped. "Well, you're lucky," he said, "because it can destroy you. I couldn't sleep, no appetite, lost weight. Didn't want to get out of bed in the morning. It was affecting my business. Anyway, someone said I should go see Jack, that he was a pretty good doctor. So I did.

"He had this dumpy little office over in Peace Dale. No secretary, no nurse. I was the only patient there. The place looked like it needed a coat of paint. He took my blood pressure, listened to my chest, and asked a lot of questions. I told him I wanted some kind of pill to at least help me sleep.

"Then out of the blue he asked me about the wife, how things were going there. You know, the physical stuff. I told him not great. After the third kid, it was like she felt she'd done enough for God and country. Just shut down. No interest. The honeymoon was definitely over."

Carl was the last patient of the day, and it was approaching six o'clock. I knew the nurse and secretary wanted to get home. "Excuse me, Carl," I said. "Let me close the place down. But don't leave – I want to hear the rest of the story. In fact, have a seat in the waiting room. The chairs are more comfortable."

The nurse had the exam rooms clean and ready to go for the next day. My efficient secretary had the day sheet with the day's cash and checks neatly bundled, and the day's dictation, excepting Carl's, all transcribed. The office phone was on answering service.

I bid them good night and rejoined Carl in the waiting room.

Carl put aside the magazine he'd been reading and continued the story. "Anyway, after Jack heard my story about the wife, he went to another room, and after five or six minutes came back. He said he wanted me to see a psychiatrist in Providence, on the East Side. 'Bullshit, Doc,' I told him. 'I just need a couple of pills. I don't want some shrink.' But Jack was adamant. He insisted. 'This man can help you,' he said. 'I'll make the arrangements and let you know where and when.'

"So, bottom line, two weeks later I saw this guy. Toney office, thick rugs, soft music. I thought to myself: The bastard's doing all right. And the guy looked like David Niven. I told him my story. He took a couple of notes but mainly just listened, nodded a couple of times like he'd heard it all before. A couple of questions about stress in my job. Then, almost as an afterthought, he asked about my sex life. 'It's lucky I have a good memory,' I told him.

"Anyway, we chatted for a while longer. Bullshit stuff. At the end of the visit he handed me a prescription. On it were two phone numbers. 'I want you to call one of these two numbers,' the doctor said, 'doesn't matter which one. A woman will answer the phone. Tell her you're a patient of mine and would like to arrange a meeting with her.'"

"Carl," I said, "you're kidding me."

"Not a word of a lie. This is exactly like it happened."

"So what did you do?"

"Called the number."

"And?"

"Within three weeks I was sleeping like a baby, energy back to normal, fun to be around, a new man."

"Depression never came back?"

"Sure, every once in a while. When it did, I just made a call. Went on for years. Phone numbers changed, but the results didn't."

"Still?"

"No, those days are long gone. But at the time it really saved my life – and my business. And the person I have to thank for it all? Jack Turco."

One afternoon approximately two years later, I received a phone call from Carl's longtime housekeeper, Marie, telling me he would like me to drop by the house after I finished in the office that afternoon.

"I will. What's going on?"

"Nothing, as far as I know. Just wanted to see you."

"Okay, tell him I'll be there about six-thirty."

"I will. I'll be gone by then. The back door will be open."

The afternoon sun was tucking into the horizon when I pulled into his driveway. A cool breeze off the water hinted of autumn. The house, a sprawling ranch, although nicely land-scaped, was of unremarkable design and size. The only hint of pretension were two white chimneys shaped like minarets, which pierced the sharp rake of a tiled roof. If it weren't for the ocean on the other side of the house, the place wouldn't have merited a second glance.

I entered through the rear of the house, announcing myself with a couple rings of the doorbell, and heard an "I'm in here" from the living room. There I found Carl seated on a couch, looking flushed. A white golf shirt with a red logo hung over baggy, wrinkled khakis. Red patches extended across his fore-head and on both cheeks.

"Sorry to waste your time, Gene, bringing you down here. But I didn't expect I'd be around when you arrived." His voice was hoarse.

"Where were you going to be?" I asked.

"Don't know." He smiled. "That's a question I've wondered all my life. You see," he continued, his tone matter-of- fact, "I just tried to commit suicide, but didn't make it. I guess you can see that."

"What in the hell are you talking about, Carl?"

He pointed to a roll of masking tape on the coffee table. A long piece had been torn off and was heaped on the floor.

"I taped my mouth and nose so air couldn't get in and just waited to die. Tried to tape my wrists so I couldn't pull it away, but couldn't manage it. So I ended up chickening out."

It was hard to tell if he was disappointed or pleased with the outcome.

"So what's up, Carl? What's going on? Why would you want to commit suicide?"

I turned on two floor lights and partially closed the drapes leading to the patio. Off in the distance, Block Island was shrouded in a luminous dusk.

"Just sick of living, I guess. You know my history, Gene. Back in the old days I used to get like this. But back then I got over it. It's different now. Can't remember for shit. Don't get around worth a damn. And I refuse to be a doddering old fool with drool dripping down my shirt. So I decided to get the whole goddamn thing over with. I've had a good enough run."

I was incredulous. He was speaking clearly, the hoarseness now gone, as if he were discussing a piece of merchandise that had passed its sell-by date and needed to be discarded. Perhaps it was a cry for help or a ploy for sympathy, but neither fit the profile of the man I knew reasonably well.

"I figured that the most efficient way to get it done," he continued, "was to call you. You'd notify the police, who would get the medical examiner. No photographers, no newspapers. I didn't want Marie to find me." He pointed to two envelopes on the coffee table. One, he said, was addressed to a local funeral director, the other to his lawyer. "Everything had been taken care of."

"You've been thinking about this for a while?"

"Yes, on and off the past few months. I'm just sorry when I finally worked up the courage I couldn't pull it off. Tried hard not to touch the tape, but finally it got so bad I pulled it off. At least it proved one thing."

"What's that?"

"That I haven't got the guts to commit suicide. That's a good thing to know." He stood and walked around the room, clearly indicating that my presence was no longer needed. The episode was over. "Anyway, I'm all right now, Gene. Sorry to drag you down here."

"You kidding me, Carl? You tell me you want to commit suicide, and then I'm supposed to leave like nothing's happened? How in the hell do I know you won't try it again? You need some help, Carl. Someone to talk with."

"No need, Gene. I promise it won't happen again. And I don't break my promises." His tone was decisive and dismissive. "I don't want any shrink calling me up." A small smile rounded the corners of his lips. "The old cure I can't do anymore."

Carl excused himself to go to the bathroom. I wondered what I should do. Absently looking around the room, I thought how much it resembled the old man. All the furniture was symmetrically arranged, each piece a monotonous beige. A single straight-backed chair sat in front of the TV. Two paintings – a landscape and a tranquil ocean scene – occupied one wall. A small desk tucked in a corner held a picture of Carl and three other men, obviously golfers, holding a trophy. No pictures of family. The decorative choices were not those of a rash personality, which made his actions this evening so out of character.

Bladder relief did nothing to change his mind regarding psychiatric intervention. My continued attempts only generated annoyance. I took my leave, with some trepidation (and the duct tape), hoping he had been scared enough not to attempt a repeat performance.

When I called his home the following morning, Marie said he was in Providence on business. He continued to visit me in the office. The home visit was never mentioned again. Carl died of natural causes four years later.

A Broken Heart

The case I remember with most clarity was a patient I acquired in 1970 from Dr. Jones, the South County physician who sent his patients to me when he retired. From our first meeting, it was evident that Belle Knowles (name altered) had weathered her seventy-five years well. Although her print dress was taut about the midsection, she carried her girth gracefully. Her face, absent makeup, was unlined; her gray hair, pulled into a bun, was encircled by flowers. Her smile seldom broadened to laughter, but blue eyes, clearly inclined to mischief, made amends.

Belle's history offered little of consequence. Her medications were of the over-the-counter variety. Absent significant complaints, I scheduled her return for four months.

As Belle maintained visits through months that became years, snippets of small talk revealed her background. Born in West Kingston, one of three siblings (all deceased), her father had been a farmer, her mother a seamstress. Her husband, John, also a farmer, had been her high school sweetheart. Regrettably, having no children was their greatest disappointment. Only Elsie, a niece who lived an hour away, visited occasionally.

"It's lonesome at times," Belle allowed. "But we have each other," was a recurring comment during our chats.

Much of their farm, originally fifteen acres, had been sold to maintain income. Belle operated a roadside vegetable stand which did a modest business. Her Christmas gifts to me were vegetables preserved in Bell jars from the summer past.

During a humid spell in August of 1973, Belle was working in the kitchen when she heard their dog barking by the barn. The barking persisted. Belle decided to investigate. When she entered the barn, John lay spread-eagled on a mound of hay, pitchfork by his side.

My condolences were received with a quiet, "thank you." Nothing else was said.

A few days later I called Elsie to ensure that Belle kept her scheduled appointment.

"Of course," she replied, then added, "It's strange, Doctor. She's acting as though nothing happened. Not a tear; never mentions John. I've tried to get her to talk..."

At the visit, Belle presented in her usual manner, with no complaints. But it soon became apparent that it was a façade, a Hollywood movie set with no one inside. Gone were the mischievous eyes; no sly smile disturbed the mask-like blankness of her face. The Belle of old was missing, buried somewhere deep inside.

"Take care of yourself, Belle," I said. "Any problem, call me. Otherwise, see you in a month."

She turned toward me. "I won't be seeing you again."

"What do you mean?"

Belle beckoned me toward her. The lips that grazed my cheek were cold. "Good-bye. Thank you."

Before I could respond, she was out the door.

By day's end, the episode, though disquieting, seemed less portentous. Naturally Belle would be depressed. But with time, I assured myself, acceptance would evolve and she would emerge from the cocoon of her grief.

I was wrong. Four days later, Elsie called to tell me that Belle had died. She was found in her parlor by the man hired to do chores. The man said that next to Belle on the couch was John and Belle's wedding picture.

Some weeks later, Elsie stopped by for a chat. Her conclusion regarding Belle: "She died of a broken heart. Pure and simple."

"You know," I replied, "it's as good a reason as any."

"Before I forget, I have something for you." She handed me a brown paper bag. "I was cleaning out Belle's pantry..."

Inside was a jar of tomatoes. The affixed square of paper read: "Save for Dr. McKee." Something in the simplicity of the gesture, the thoughtfulness, caught me off guard. After a mumbled, "Thanks, must get back to work," I turned away.

> In 1991 Japanese cardiologists reported a series of unusual cases. The patients, primarily post-menopausal women, presented with signs and symptoms (often minimal) of heart attack; their electrocardiograms and lab data were not consistent with the diagnosis. Examination of heart vessels indicated no significant disease or blockage. Common to all was physical or emotional stress immediately prior to the event.
>
> The condition's cause was thought to be a surge of stress hormones, the precise mechanism unclear. What is known: the heart muscle is stunned to the extent that efficient circulation cannot be maintained. Attempting to compensate, a portion of the heart enlarges, assuming the shape of a pot used in Japan to trap octopus – initially it was called "takotsubo" disease. As cases were reported worldwide, it became known as broken-heart syndrome. With prompt recognition and treatment, the prognosis is good.

Elsie's intuition eight years earlier was spot on. Interestingly, the following appears in Shakespeare's *Macbeth* (1606):

> *"Give sorrow words;*
> *the grief that does not speak*
> *whispers the o'er fraught heart*
> *and bids it break."*

Lights Out

My final day practicing medicine, forty-four years after Mary Tafuri cashed my check, occurred on the last day of January, 2013.

The urgent care staff had hosted a going-away party for me at a local restaurant two weeks earlier, not wanting to take any chances that I might change my mind. All wished me a happy and healthy retirement. The murmurs of "Thank God," I chose to ignore.

The evening did have moments of second guessing as they were a great group to work with. But as with similar decisions over the years, a certainty had developed, and I knew it was time to go. Another consideration: I would be leaving with my apron clean, free of malpractice stains – and I wanted to keep it that way.

The last physician I had the pleasure of working with was Dr. Carla Cesario, our own *Little Mary Sunshine.*

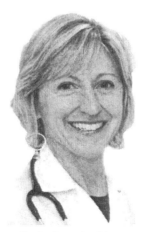

Carla Cesario, M.D.

Energetic, consistently pleasant, with an impressive clinical knowledge and extraordinary patient rapport, she kept me on my toes over the last two years. Her services were so well thought of that, unlike her older colleague, she regularly received thank-you notes and gift cards to fancy restaurants from grateful patients. Certainly well-deserved, but the flaunting of her culinary coup the following day – how the Riesling paired well with the caviar – was cruel. Nevertheless, if she is the face of the current crop of primary care physicians, we are in good shape.

The Passing Decades

As I recall the years, I feel fortunate to have worked in what I consider one of the most extraordinary eras in American medicine. The transformation of the profession from the mid-1960s through the turn of the century could be compared to the journey from the Dark Ages to the Age of Enlightenment.

South County Hospital was a microcosm of this transition. In 1965 it was a bare-bones institution, as many were at that time. The hospital boasted fourteen doctors on staff; antibiotics were the new kids on the block; diagnostic modalities were limited to lab, X-ray, and a borrowed EKG machine.

Then came the 1970s, with an influx of physicians representing all specialties; at the end of that decade forty physicians comprised the staff. A meager pharmacopeia was energized and included: angiotension converting enzyme (ACE inhibitors) and calcium channel blockers (CCB) for hypertension, the statins as lipid inhibitors, and selective serotonin reuptake inhibitors (SSRI's) for depression.

With each successive decade the advance continued: the 1980s brought the CAT scan and laser eye surgery, the 1990s MRI, laparoscopic gall bladder surgery, angioplasty, and stent placement (non-cardiac), birthing rooms, on-campus radiation therapy, and a multitude of out-patient services.

The new century saw an increase of interventional radiological procedures, with laparoscopic and robotic surgeries becoming commonplace. A recent (2016) hospital out-reach has been the palliative care program. A multi-disciplinary effort, it provides a coordinated support system to address the physical and psychosocial needs of the ill patient to improve quality of life.

Likewise, the development of the physical plant has been impressive: structurally and aesthetically. The imposing hospital that sat grandly on an elevated stretch of land in 1970 has been subsumed into administrative space: a series of offices strung along corridors buffed to a gleam, the hum of activity behind closed doors the only sound. Not a hint of the bustle, the throb of activity, the antiseptic smell, the daily dramas, that filled that space not so long ago.

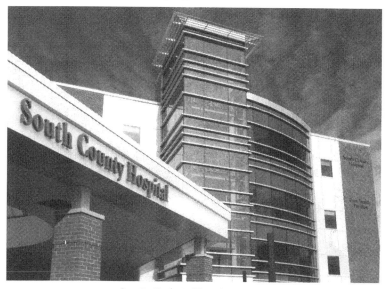

South County Hospital, 2016

In its stead, a gleaming edifice towers over an attractive campus and acres of parking, which on most days are filled with cars, a measure of the myriad and well-attended services offered. When I see this abundance of activity and the sprawling, splendid architecture, I am struck by the fact that it's still a one hundred-bed hospital, the same as it was when I first walked through its doors in 1970. The parking space necessary then was the lot on the Kenyon Avenue side of the hospital. An apples and oranges comparison for sure but I think it inter-esting that the level of in-patient activity – has not changed in forty-five years.

Recruitment of physicians has kept pace. There are cur-rently (2016), forty-seven physicians and fourteen mid-level providers on staff in the South County Medical Group, a part of South County Health (the name change meant to encompass the broad sweep of health services offered to the community).

Some physicians employed by the hospital are just beginning their practice. The benefits of this arrangement are mutual: the utilization of hospital services by the physician and a degree of financial stability for the doctors building their patient base. I remember well my concerns when I started practice and how I would have welcomed such an arrangement.

Another physician option not present in "the day," are hos-pitalists: well-trained physicians who assume care of a majority of the hospitalized medical patients – a luxury I can't imagine. The most demanding work of medicine, I believe, was caring for in-patients. The initial intervention (usually in the emer-gency room), the phone calls, nighttime visits, daily rounds, and anxiety attached to patients not doing well, could be trying. To have that responsibility assumed by someone else would have been tempting.

The possible downside: A practice confined to an office can, over time, allow a laxity to develop, a procrastination to staying current, a gradual slide into auto-pilot mode.

In the hospital setting you have to be at the top of your game. It requires an effort to think more, read more, discuss and learn more from other physicians and the nurses. To lose this stimulation in return for a more comfortable lifestyle (which I probably would have done) is a questionable trade-off.

In this day of conglomerate acquisition, South County remains the only independent hospital in the state of Rhode Island. And in a miracle of management alchemy, the institution's finances, as of 2015, have run in the black for the past five years.

Nor is it resting on its laurels, as it extends its brand and services: an Urgent Care Center in East Greenwich and most recently, the Medical and Wellness Center in Westerly, Rhode Island. They are moves that will have South County Hospital nicely positioned to be the major health player in southern Rhode Island.

Lou Giancola, the hospital's president and CEO, as well as his talented team and innovative board of trustees, deserve a prolonged round of applause.

A Nice Touch

Some observers would argue that the changes in medicine have not all been positive, that the relationship and rapport between physician and patient have been diminished by a ubiquitous technology.

My friend "Ted," recently decided the time had come for a physical exam. He had some nagging physical issues he wanted to put to rest. A call was made to an internist who could see Ted in four weeks.

The office was nicely appointed, the exam room bright and clean, with a selection of current magazines in the wall rack.

After a brief introduction, a series of questions were directed toward him from a nurse (he presumed), hunched over a laptop. His answers were nimbly transcribed onto a multicolored screen. After the young lady massaged a disinfectant into her hands, vital signs were taken. A machine displayed his blood pressure and pulse; a swipe of an instrument across his forehead read his temperature. The nurse's hand briefly grazed his when she removed the blood pressure cuff.

The interaction with the physician included a detailed past history discussion and an informative conversation regarding Ted's medical concerns, at the end of which, chest X-rays and an ultrasound were scheduled for later in the week. Lab requisition slips were obtained as was the phone number of a urologist. The doctor never touched the patient.

Although the laying on of hands may arguably be of little value and the stethoscope less a diagnostic tool than a totem of authority, the gentleman who described this encounter mentioned – with some sarcasm – that the use of either, although "quaint," would have been a "nice touch." He also agreed with me that his experience was probably an anomaly, but he wondered if it could be a hint of the future.

It brings to mind the current concerns of some airlines: pilots who have forgotten how to fly planes manually. Once the flight plan is fed into the computer, today's aviators basically become observers, tweaking the computer as necessary to avoid bad weather or as advised by ground control. These high-speed, high-altitude gamers may have to figure out how to land the aircraft when the screen goes dark, and some have little idea. The comparison between the two occupations may be faulty – although both deal with the lives of others – but it does illustrate how wed to technology we've become.

Patients have also changed. When I was growing up, the dictates of both priest and doctor bordered on infallibility. If the diagnosis of rheumatic fever in a young person was deemed by the family doctor to require six months in bed, that was the end of the conversation. Not true today, which is a good thing; people are better informed. And they are not shy about presenting information to the doctor, gleaned from any number of sources. Most physicians, including myself, enjoy the ensuing interchanges, especially when they result in mutual agreement.

In our urgent care facility, it was not unusual for patients to present with Google reprints, addressing signs and symptoms similar to theirs. Often they were spot-on, and the patients were pleased with their insight. Others, however, wouldn't accept the physician's opinion. "My cousin or (fill in the blank) says I have the same thing they had, and it's not what you're telling me." Soon the cell phone came out, and the patient discussed the situation with the relative or friend. If the impasse continued, the relationship deteriorated, leaving in its wake a frustrated physician and an angry patient who would "check with my own doctor in the morning," and who left, often without paying the bill.

This scenario is something of an exception, but it's an exception encountered more often than you might imagine.

A Noble Endeavor

I have been asked on occasion if I was sorry that I didn't enter a specialty field. My answer was that I did enter a specialty field – family medicine, a discipline whose spectrum of care happens to be wider than others. My first board exam was in 1972 with re-certifications every seven years, the last in 2009. Over the course of my career in medicine, I have enjoyed a breadth of activities and roles: aviation and industrial medicine, quality assurance, acute care, school and athletic physician. I don't think those opportunities would have been offered if my focus had been narrowed to a particular field.

I'm of the school that prefers to know a little bit about a lot of things rather than the converse. The variety of patients and pathologies one sees in a busy family practice is one of its attractions.

The most daunting task for a physician, I feel, is living up to the trust patients place in you. A bumper sticker I saw years ago read, "I want to be the man my dog thinks I am." The same could apply to medicine, to be the doctor the patient thinks you are.

Over the years I've taken care of hundreds of families, stretching over generations, who put their faith in my ability to handle their medical needs. For decades they believed I would do the right thing for them. That's a scary responsibility: not to do harm or let down those who have trusted you for so long. Possibly at some subconscious level, beyond the exotic continuing medical education destinations and medical licensure mandates, that is the reason physicians make the effort to stay current in their field.

The existence of this physician/patient dynamic barely crossed my mind while in active practice. Only when the positions were reversed, and I or a family member had to trust that the physician was as good as his dog thought he was, did I more fully appreciate that someone once had the same confidence in me.

The practice of medicine has always been, and I'm confident always will be, a noble endeavor. Delivery systems and treatments will continue to evolve, but for the foreseeable future, it will continue to be an interaction between two people, one of whom is able to help the other. I applaud and endorse the changes, as Dr. Jones did forty years ago. The advances made during my brief career have been of the mind-boggling variety; the pocket-size Merck Manual I lugged around during my training days is now, many revised editions later, etched onto a chip in my cell phone.

That doesn't mean, however, that you never miss the pre-binary days, which for most emeritus-designated physicians seems a simpler, more ordinary time. Just as lilting melodies, intelligible lyrics, ballroom dancing, and movies where the promise of sex was found in the nuance of a glance are but nostalgic artifacts, so too are many of the rituals familiar to the graying physician...gone the way of "wet" x-ray readings and Blakemore tubes. And, of course, that's as it should be.

The exercise of putting together a memoir allows one to relish the life you have been privileged to enjoy, which for the most part has been taken for granted. But rooting around the nooks and crannies, you come across — along with the champagne and glad days — the beer and bad days, repressed and tucked away in the closet of memory. Like torn theater stubs discovered in the folds of an old tuxedo, they remind that life, like the stage, has its share of conflict and complications – and every play has a third act for a reason.

The criteria which I believe offer the definition of a successful medical career: you have gained the respect of peers and those you've worked with; in your care of patients you have done more good than harm; and you have made enough money to afford a decent nursing home.

In my conceit, I feel I have met the first two requirements. The third is less certain. But as the singer Meat Loaf advised back in the '70s:

"Now don't be sad
'Cause two out of three ain't bad"

E. B. McKee, M.D.

About the Author

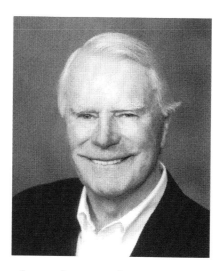

After graduation from the Royal College of Surgeons in 1961, Dr. McKee completed an internship and residency in Family Medicine at Memorial Hospital in Pawtucket R.I. Then, fulfilling an ROTC commitment, he entered the US Air Force, and was assigned to the 551st USAF Hospital at Otis AFB on Cape Cod, Mass., as a General Medical Officer. Subsequently he was chosen to attend the School of Aerospace Medicine in San Antonio, Texas.

Upon completion of that program he returned to Otis AFB where he headed the Flight Surgeons office. Discharged from active military duty in 1966, he joined the medical staff of United Airlines working in Denver; Washington, D.C.; and New York. (Dr. McKee maintained a military affiliation and retired, after twenty years of service, as Hospital Commander of the 143rd Airlift Wing, R. I. Air National Guard.)

Dr. McKee returned to R.I. in 1970 and established a family practice, became board-certified, and maintained the practice until 2000. During this time-span he also directed the occupational health program at the Electric Boat Division of General Dynamics in R.I.

Dr. McKee occupied a number of executive and clinical leadership positions at South County Hospital in Wakefield, R.I., and has enjoyed associations with various medical and civic organizations over the years. He is a member of the R.I. Air National Guard Society, Mensa, and the R.I. Historical Society.

Dr. McKee was appointed Medical Director of an urgent care facility, a position he maintained until his retirement in 2013.

Married and the father of five, Dr. McKee presently resides in Narragansett, R.I. Author contact: genem1@cox.net

Also read McKee's memoir:

DOC

How a Reluctant Yank Found Himself Becoming a Physician Among the Irish

Prodded by his formidable Aunt Bertha to become a doctor, college-grad, Gene McKee, agrees to explore Europe in search of a welcoming medical school. Seizing the opportunity will provide relief from the tedium and stench of a temporary job as a fish cutter in Rhode Island.

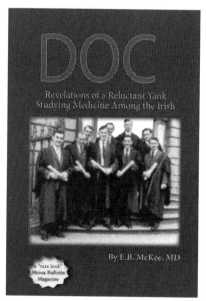

The frustrations and apparent futility of the quest, extending through Ireland, England, Scotland, and France, test his resolve. But just before the clock's final tick, an unlikely acceptance to the Royal College of Surgeons in Dublin opens the door to a future not exactly of his own choosing.

McKee's rite-of-passage travelogue is replete with anecdotes of medical school and Dublin life during the late 1950s and early 60s. Recounted with self-deprecating humor and considerable honesty, we witness McKee's transformation from a reluctant medical student to a competent physician. Enjoyably peppered with historical tidbits, amorous entanglements, and imaginative riffs, reading *DOC* and seeing Ireland with its rich cast of "characters" through a young Irish-American's eyes, will surely bring smiles to the faces of readers and for some, a twinge of recognition.

DOC is available from Amazon, Barnes & Noble and from local bookstores everywhere.

Made in the USA
Charleston, SC
22 February 2017